AF818011

Secondary Trauma

Robert W. Motta

# Secondary Trauma

## Silent Suffering and Its Treatment

Springer

Robert W. Motta
Department of Psychology
Hofstra University
Hempstead, NY, USA

ISBN 978-3-031-44307-7 ISBN 978-3-031-44308-4 (eBook)
https://doi.org/10.1007/978-3-031-44308-4

© The Editor(s) (if applicable) and The Author(s), under exclusive license to Springer Nature Switzerland AG 2023
This work is subject to copyright. All rights are solely and exclusively licensed by the Publisher, whether the whole or part of the material is concerned, specifically the rights of translation, reprinting, reuse of illustrations, recitation, broadcasting, reproduction on microfilms or in any other physical way, and transmission or information storage and retrieval, electronic adaptation, computer software, or by similar or dissimilar methodology now known or hereafter developed.
The use of general descriptive names, registered names, trademarks, service marks, etc. in this publication does not imply, even in the absence of a specific statement, that such names are exempt from the relevant protective laws and regulations and therefore free for general use.
The publisher, the authors, and the editors are safe to assume that the advice and information in this book are believed to be true and accurate at the date of publication. Neither the publisher nor the authors or the editors give a warranty, expressed or implied, with respect to the material contained herein or for any errors or omissions that may have been made. The publisher remains neutral with regard to jurisdictional claims in published maps and institutional affiliations.

This Springer imprint is published by the registered company Springer Nature Switzerland AG
The registered company address is: Gewerbestrasse 11, 6330 Cham, Switzerland

Paper in this product is recyclable.

*This work is dedicated to my wife, Teresa. Her inspiration and support have been foundational in bringing this work to fruition.*

# Introduction

This book is intended to increase the understanding of the concept of secondary trauma and its treatment. Secondary trauma and secondary traumatic stress disorder (STSD) refer to the emotional upset one experiences in response to the distress encountered by others. The notion that the distress of others could lead to emotional disruption in those who care for, or are involved with that person or persons, was popularized by Charles Figley (1995) and was often referred to as "compassion fatigue" (p. 1), but it is not a novel concept. The economist Adam Smith wrote of the reactions to the distress of others as early as 1759. For example, taking care of a family member who is coping with a serious medical or psychological condition can result in emotional turmoil and exhaustion in the caretaker. The caretaker's distress is but one example of a secondary trauma. Another example might be that of firefighters, police officers, EMTs, and other frontline workers who attempt to help those in crisis and who then acquire emotional distress as an outcome of their witnessing the pain of those they are trying to assist. The spouse of a combat veteran who has been diagnosed with PTSD might develop symptoms that look much like PTSD. A final example is that of the psychotherapist whose caseload is composed primarily of highly traumatized individuals such as those who have been physically or sexually assaulted. After listening for many hours to details of such assaults, the therapist begins to become wary and anxious around people who might bear any similarity to the described attackers. The therapist's thoughts and dreams might encompass images of abuse and they might begin to develop panic and other unexplained fear responses. The therapist might begin to doubt the security and safety of their environment. All of these are examples of what is referred to in the literature by terms such as secondary traumatic stress disorder (STSD), burnout, secondary trauma, vicarious trauma, or "compassion fatigue" (Figley, 1995). Regardless of the terms that are used, these people suffer in silence. They shoulder the burdens of others and often do so without complaint.

Given the variety of terms describing secondary trauma and given the wide array of instances in which secondary trauma might occur, certain guidelines will be adhered to in this book to provide structure and clarity. The first is that secondary trauma will be used as a generic term to apply to instances in which distress is transferred from one person or persons to others primarily as a function of one or more individuals caring for, supporting, or attending to others. The interchangeability of terms such as vicarious traumatization, secondary traumatic stress, empathic strain, and compassion fatigue has precedent in the literature (e.g., Phipps & Byrne, 2003; Sexton, 1999). The next guideline to be followed will be that the *primary* sources of secondary trauma occur in situations involving (a) *the family*, that is, one or more family members caring for a traumatized, physically ill, or emotionally troubled family member or members; (b) *professional caregivers*, that is, situations in which a therapist, medical doctor, nurse, or other health-care provider becomes emotionally depleted or otherwise distressed because of the incapacitation, illness, injury, or emotional distress of a person or persons that the professional care provider is treating; and (c) *first responders*, that is, firefighters, police officers, EMTs, paramedics, disaster response workers, and other community helpers whose job entails the provision and overseeing of public safety, security, and well-being. These individuals can become emotionally overwhelmed or depleted because of the demanding nature of their jobs and the witnessing of the trauma and distress of others.

There are many other circumstances and occupations where secondary trauma might occur such as insurance claims adjusters, librarians, or pharmacists who are desperately called upon to provide information or other support for those in distress (Figley & Ludick, 2017) and even in those who are engaged in foster care (Hannah & Woolgar, 2018). In fact, Motta (2015, p. 68) includes a partial listing of situations in which secondary trauma has been investigated including in family members (Catherall, 1992), in partners of those who have been abused (Nelson & Wampler, 2000), in wives of combat veterans with PTSD (Waysman et al., 1993), in adult children of Vietnam veterans with PTSD (Suozzi & Motta, 2004), in wives of police officers (Dwyer, 2005), in grandchildren of Holocaust survivors (Kassai & Motta, 2006; Kellerman, 2001; Perlstein & Motta, 2012), in family members of those with a serious medical illness (Boyer et al., 2002; Libov et al., 2002; Lombardo, 2005), and in children of parents with mental illness (Lombardo, 2007). Gilbert-Eliot (2020, pp. 4–7) includes law enforcement workers, firefighters, paramedics, emergency medical technicians, mental health therapists, emergency room staff, child welfare workers, spouses and family members of people in trauma-prone professions, and caregivers of someone with a serious medical issue, and states, "That's not an exhaustive list" (p. 7). However, in the interest of clarity and focus and in consideration of the fact that the major thrust of the literature is seen in the three areas above, that is, in families, in professional caregivers, and in first responders, these will be the primary areas of focus in this book.

## Diagnostic Overlap

Secondary trauma is not as precisely defined as post-traumatic stress disorder (PTSD) in the current version of the *Diagnostic and Statistical Manual of Mental Disorders* (fifth ed. [*DSM-5*]; American Psychiatric Association, 2013). In fact, secondary trauma is not a diagnostic category in the *DSM*. Nevertheless, *The Secondary Trauma Scale* (Motta et al., 1999, 2001) provides cutoff scores for diagnosing secondary trauma and provides descriptors such as intrusive thoughts and avoidance behaviors. Additionally, there can be overlap between PTSD and secondary trauma, and this can create confusion in understanding the two terms. For example, the police, firefighters, and other first responders who frequently witness the distress of others are often diagnosed as having been secondarily traumatized, but they can also develop PTSD. In the *DSM-5*, we find the following listed among the diagnostic features of PTSD: "Witnessed events include … observing threatened or serious injury … physical or sexual abuse of another person due to violent assault, domestic violence … or a medical catastrophe in one's own child (e.g., a life-threatening hemorrhage)" (p. 274). The point being made here is that there are times when first responders might be exposed to the observance of "threatened or serious injury." These instances might then become potential stressors leading to PTSD. A recent book by Bryant (2021) specifically addresses PTSD and its treatment in first responders. In the absence of PTSD, however, when their daily obligations and routines to assure the safety of others become emotionally draining, then a diagnosis of secondary traumatization might be more appropriate. Despite this potential diagnostic overlap, in general PTSD is most often associated with serious personal threats and extreme fears, while secondary trauma is the acquisition of emotional distress arising from close association and involvement with others who are traumatized.

## Activities Associated with Secondary Trauma

In addition to the categories noted above that are sources of secondary trauma, a partial listing of *activities* from which secondary trauma might arise is provided by Gilbert-Eliot (2020). These activities include those of law enforcement workers, firefighters, paramedics and EMTs, mental health therapists, emergency room staff, child welfare workers, spouses, and other family members of people in trauma-producing professions, and caregivers of someone with a serious medical condition (pp. 4–5). A good deal of the existing literature on secondary traumatization has to do with the negative impact on health-care providers that occurs in response to working with trauma victims. This major focus on the distress of health-care workers seems to be due to the fact that the secondary trauma literature is often produced by those with some association with the health-care field, including psychotherapists, physicians, occupational therapists, nurses, and rehabilitation specialists. However, most secondary trauma episodes have little to do with health-care providers and far more to do with family members or close friends who are negatively impacted by their association with an emotionally or physically traumatized individual or individuals (National Alliance for Caregiving [NAC], 2020).

This situation, where the knowledge base regarding secondary trauma is derived from health-care provider experiences rather than family members, is like that of

PTSD where the knowledge base is derived from studies of military combatants. But surprisingly, military experiences represent a comparatively small source of actual PTSD cases. Most of the PTSD diagnoses arise from distress originating in the civilian world. There are far more cases of PTSD due to rapes, assaults, various forms of child abuse, spousal maltreatment, extreme financial hardships, life-threatening ailments, auto accidents, natural disasters, and other civilian experiences than there are from the military. This in no way trivializes the potential negative impact of military experience but rather highlights that a comparatively small percentage of PTSD diagnoses arise from combat simply because there are far fewer people involved in military conflicts in comparison to civilians who encounter a wide range of traumas. Similarly, most secondary trauma cases evolve from experiencing the distress of family members and friends rather than the distress of health-care providers or first responders. The major sources of trauma, whether primary, as in PTSD, or secondary, occur among those who are noncombatants and non-frontline personnel.

Secondary traumatization, unlike PTSD, is the negative emotional, physical, and perhaps spiritually negative state that occurs in people who work with those who are in distress, such as those who are enduring a traumatic experience, including PTSD. Those suffering PTSD have encountered primary traumatic experiences and react with extreme fear. In contrast, those with secondary trauma are negatively impacted by their involvement with a primary trauma sufferer. The person experiencing secondary trauma will often feel that their ability to cope has been compromised and as a result feel overwhelmed. They are burdened, sullen, and often despairing and yet they often bear their burdens in silence. In many ways, they have been emotionally impacted by, and carry the burdens of, a person or persons who have experienced primary trauma. However, describing secondary trauma and PTSD as highly similar is unjustified. "Compassion Fatigue is a more user friendly term for Secondary Traumatic Stress Disorder, which is nearly identical to PTSD …" (Figley, 2003, p. 3). Despite this statement, these two concepts are dissimilar in terms of etiology, symptomology, and treatment. The concept of "emotional contagion" (Hatfield et al., 1994) or the spreading of emotions from one to another is a good descriptor of what takes place in secondary traumatization but not in PTSD.

## Related Terms

As noted previously, there appear to be several terms, all of which are relevant to the negative impact that is encountered when one is exposed to, and perhaps must deal with, traumatized individuals and environments. For example, vicarious traumatization, a concept coined by McCann and Pearlman (1990), refers to the transformation of health workers' inner experience following the conducting of extensive trauma therapy sessions. This transformation includes alterations in one's sense of meaning, connection, identity, and work experiences, as well as "one's affect tolerance, psychological needs, beliefs about self and others, interpersonal relationships, and sensory memory, including imagery" (Pearlman & Saakvitne, 1995, p. 151). "Compassion fatigue," similarly, reflects the emotional drain and depletion resulting from working with those who are traumatized (Figley, 1995, p. 1). A related term, "empathy-based stress" (Rauvola et al., 2019) is also used synonymously with compassion fatigue.

Burnout, a term initially presented by Freudenberger (1974) and fully explicated by Maslach (1976), is applicable to work environments, often those environments involving the providing of assistance to health-impaired individuals, that results in the worker's feeling of emotional exhaustion and demoralization. These work environments might be counseling centers, schools for those with handicapping conditions, hospitals, and so on. However, burnout need not be the result of working with people. Exhausting and emotionally draining labor of any kind might be the cause of burnout. Another area where the term burnout has been applied is with families experiencing secondary trauma; see, for example, *Burnout in families: The systematic costs of caring* (Figley, 1998). Emotional contagion (Hatfield, 1994), although not necessarily trauma-specific, refers more broadly to the tendency to be influenced by and "feel" the emotionality of others. The term secondary traumatic stress disorder (STSD; Figley, 1995) is also of relevance here and is described below in the treatment section.

Despite definitional nuances that arise from, and seem related to, the source of the secondary traumatic experience, there is no widely agreed-upon and empirically validated differentiation among these various terms. One of the few exceptions is that of Adams et al. (2008) who found that among social workers involved with the September 11, 2001, attack on the World Trade Center in New York, exposure to traumatized patients increased vicarious trauma but not job burnout. In turn, both vicarious trauma and job burnout were related to the experiencing of psychological problems. But in general, both burnout and secondary trauma involve an emotional depletion that occurs because of giving of oneself and both are associated with psychological adjustment difficulties. For this reason, the various terms including "secondary traumatization," "secondary trauma," "vicarious trauma," and others will be used in this book to describe the transfer of emotional distress from one individual to another regardless of the context in which this transfer occurs.

## Trauma Treatment

In addition to misconceptions about the major sources of, and differences between, primary and secondary trauma, there appears to be some confusion regarding how to deal with trauma, whether primary or secondary. Many of our trauma interventions are heavily influenced by a medical model that emphasizes "diseases," "illnesses," "treatments," and "cures," and this emphasis becomes a source of potential confusion in our investigation of secondary trauma. This medically derived mode of reasoning has had an impact on the world of psychotherapy where we encounter terms such as mental "illness," "chemical imbalances," "treatments," and the need for "psychotropic medications." It is not that serious mental disturbances don't exist. They do and they create significant pain for all who are involved. And it is true that medication can be of value in treating some of the more serious disorders such as schizophrenia, bipolar disorder, and obsessive-compulsive disorder. Medical intervention is of substantial benefit in these cases but the prevalence of these disorders in the general population is small and ranges from approximately 1–3% for each (Jamison, 1999). These "illnesses" are doubtlessly serious and are damaging to well-being, but most psychological problems are not medically based illnesses. Rather, they are problems that are encountered by those who are having difficulty coping with distressing experiences and problematic environments. Secondary traumatization is this type of problem. Figley (1995, p. 8), for example, describes the condition of secondary traumatic stress disorder (STSD) in the following way:

> A syndrome of symptoms nearly identical to PTSD [post-traumatic stress disorder], except that exposure to knowledge about a traumatizing event experienced by a significant other is associated with the set of STSD symptoms, and PTSD symptoms are directly connected to the sufferer, the person experiencing primary traumatic stress.

STSD is not an illness but a form of emotional distress for which several practical, nonmedical interventions are helpful. While Figley's (1995) definition does not imply that the condition of STSD is a medical problem, paradoxically, an aspect of medical terminology can be helpful in grasping a problem like secondary trauma. For example, some medical illnesses are contagious such as flu or the highly communicable COVID-19 virus. The contagious nature of viruses helps us in understanding secondary trauma. Trauma can be said to be "contagious" in so far as it involves the transfer of emotional pain from the sufferer to the observer. The observer can be a family member, close friend, frontline worker, or health-care member. Caring for others can sometimes result in being "infected" by their pain. This "infection" is what characterizes secondary trauma regardless of the definitional nuances in some of the terms that are used. Because secondary traumatization is the negative emotional, physical, and perhaps spiritually negative state that occurs in people who work with those who are in distress, such as those who are going through a traumatic experience, it can come across as being contagious. Thus, while medical model conceptualizations of trauma and the transfer of trauma reactions may not accurately reflect what is taking place, they can serve as a way of grasping the contagious nature of trauma.

The various "treatments" for secondary trauma are oriented toward easing or lessening the impact of this psychological stressor. Many interventions involve life adjustments and alterations, such as maintaining balance in one's personal life and using personal and group therapy (Norcross, 2000; Pearlman & Saakvitne, 1995). The use of meditation, yoga, exercise, interaction with animals, and outdoor environments have also shown themselves to be of value at least as far as managing PTSD is concerned (Benedek & Wynn, 2016; Motta, 2020) and would presumably be beneficial for secondary trauma. Despite theoretical claims and convictions, there is little empirical support for the notion that there exists specified individual or group therapy interventions that are demonstrably better or more effective than others and this is true for both primary and secondary trauma. The current widely accepted view is that the best mode of treatment for PTSD, a primary trauma, is cognitive-behavioral psychotherapy. "The treatment of choice for PTSD … is exposure based cognitive therapy" (Preston et al., 2002, p. 137). However, when one digs into the literature to examine double-blind, placebo-controlled studies with random assignment, there is no universal support for this position. Wompold et al. (2010), for example, following extensive meta-analyses, maintained that it is the therapeutic relationship that is beneficial and curative, and the impact of specific therapeutic techniques is comparatively less important.

If we are uncertain regarding the most effective treatment for PTSD, then we are even more unaware of the best treatment for secondary traumas as these sorts of traumas are far less researched than PTSD (Maynard & Bercer, 2015). Given the relative lack of knowledge regarding secondary trauma treatment, there is little reason to believe that interventions that have proven valuable in treating primary trauma and PTSD would or would not be useful in treating secondary traumatization. In a thorough review of studies relevant to the treatment of compassion fatigue (CF), secondary traumatic stress (STS), and vicarious trauma (VT), Bercier & Maynard (2015, p. 87) conclude, "While there may be some aspects or techniques of primary trauma treatment that can inform and be adapted to treat CF, STS, and VT, we should be careful to not assume that trauma interventions intended to treat primary trauma will be effective in treating CF, STS, and VT." In fact, in their review they found virtually no treatments for secondary trauma that were empirically supported as being better than others and as a result they found no data-based conclusions regarding treatment efficacy for secondary trauma. So, in addition to delving into various issues related to secondary trauma, this book will examine various treatment approaches that might be of value in its treatment. A particular emphasis will be placed on nontraditional treatments. Nontraditional treatments refer to interventions that do not follow traditional models of treatment such as CBT, behavioral therapy, analytic procedures, and the like. This emphasis on nontraditional treatment is chosen for three reasons. First, there is little evidence to suggest that those suffering from secondary trauma have the cognitive misconceptions or errors in thinking that point to the selection of CBT or other traditional treatments. These cognitive misconceptions are a principal target of cognitive-behavioral psychotherapy. Rather, those with secondary trauma appear to be experiencing a somewhat expected kind of distress and emotional depletion that results from working with distressed individuals. Their reactions are generally not psychopathological or irrational and therefore traditional forms of therapy may not be needed. Second, nontraditional treatment interventions such as yoga, meditation, and exercise are often less intrusive than traditional CBT treatments are as a result are less likely to be avoided (Motta, 2020) by those suffering from secondary trauma. And finally, the alternatives to traditional treatments that are presented are those that have received some degree of empirical support at least as far as treating PTSD is concerned, and this support usually comes through controlled studies or metanalyses, or both.

## Chapter Overview

Many actual case examples are provided throughout this book. Case names, localities, professions, and other possibly identifying information have been altered to maintain confidentiality. Nevertheless, the essential aspects of these cases have been maintained to be as close to reality as possible while not risking the possibility of identification of those involved. The only exception is when a well-known case that has already been publicized in the media is being presented.

The origins of the development of secondary trauma and empathy are covered in Chap. 1. Here, it is shown that empathy in humans develops at a very early age. It is also shown that empathic and compassionate responding is not uniquely human but is shown by primates and other animals. The evolutionary advantage of empathy and secondary trauma is highlighted. The role of "mirror neurons" is also addressed. Chapter 2 continues to trace the evolution of secondary trauma by highlighting secondary trauma in childhood and the overarching importance of loss of attachments in children's lives. Chapter 3 addresses the most common sources of secondary trauma and consequent emotional exhaustion, namely that which occurs when members of a family must attend to and care for another member who might be seriously physically ill or emotionally distressed. Chapter 4 focuses on professional caregivers such as psychotherapists, physicians, nurses, and physician assistants. An important element in the development of PTSD and secondary trauma is highlighted, namely the perceived inability to escape one's professional demands and obligations. In Chap. 5, there is a presentation of the unique stressors experienced by first responders such as police officers, firefighters, EMTs, paramedics, and disaster relief workers. The role of personality characteristics and how those characteristics play into the development of secondary trauma is addressed. Chapter 6 examines considerations for treating STSD and contrasts such treatment with what might be provided in cases of PTSD. Some authors claim that STSD and PTSD are nearly identical and that their treatment is also highly similar. The chapter highlights the actual dissimilarities between PTSD and STSD and questions the need for similarities in treatment. Chapter 7 deals with structural interventions for secondary trauma. These are pragmatic intervention strategies that focus on the restructuring of work activities and the seeking out of self-care activities. Structural interventions are contrasted with traditional, individually administered therapeutic approaches such as those employed in CBT. Chapter 8 highlights the important role of social support in lessening the negative consequences of secondary trauma within families, among first responders, and in professional care providers. It also investigates those factors that might mitigate the utility of social support. Chapter 9 focuses on the role of physical exercise as a means of coping with and reducing the impact of secondary traumatization. Various theoretical views are presented that attempt to explain why exercise might be helpful in cases of secondary traumatization. Chapter 10 deals with the role that mindfulness meditation plays in alleviating trauma and secondary trauma symptoms. Examples of mindfulness practices are highlighted along with empirical research supporting the value of meditation in managing secondary trauma. Chapter 11 covers the increasingly popular practice of yoga as a way of dealing with life stressors including those due to secondary trauma. Reviews of the research literature are presented showing empirical support for yoga as a way of managing secondary trauma. A variety of the more popular forms of yoga practice are also presented. Chapter 12 deals with the unique role that animals play in reducing the stress levels of humans. A wide variety of animals have been identified as helpful in reducing stress of the kind found in both PTSD and secondary traumatization. Chapter 13 includes systematic studies of paraprofessional interventions and self-care strategies for managing secondary trauma. The novel and important role of natural environments as a source of secondary traumatic stress relief is also reviewed. Chapter 14 provides summary comments and observations.

# Acknowledgments

I would like to thank those associated with Springer who supported the publication of this book. Sharon Panulla in acquisitions recognized the potential value of a book on secondary trauma. Velarasu Hemalatha, Cynthia Pushparaj, and Suvedha Sivaramakrishnan are also acknowledged for their individual contributions in finalizing this work. Finally, I thank all of those whose individual and often private suffering with secondary trauma inspired the writing of this book. Special thanks to Jason, Fara, and Marsha Smith for their support in having their story told.

# Contents

# Chapter 1
# Origins

## 1.1 Where Does the Capacity for Secondary Traumatization Come from?

While there is no way of time traveling into our evolutionary past to determine where and when empathy and consequent secondary traumatization may have arisen, it is reasonable to assume that these phenomena served survival purposes in our distant past, and because of this, we may be biologically programmed to respond compassionately and be impacted by the stress that is inherent in responding compassionately. Concern for others must have had a facilitative effect on group survival and afforded an evolutionary advantage (Hoffman, 1975). An essential element of compassionate responding and therefore of secondary traumatization is empathy.

Adam Smith, the recognized father of economics in the USA and particularly the economic benefits of self-interest, defined empathy as unselfish interest in the "fortune" of others and provided the classic description of sympathy, a related and perhaps necessary component of secondary trauma and empathy, in this way: "By changing places in fancy with the sufferer, that we come either to conceive or to be affected by what he feels…" (1759/1948, p. 74). We are thus capable of feeling the pain of someone else and can react as if we too are in pain. He further wrote, "When we see a stroke aimed, and just ready to fall upon the leg or arm of another person, we naturally shrink and draw back our leg or our own arm; and when it does fall, we feel it in some measure, and are hurt by it as well as the sufferer" (Smith, 1759/1976, p. 10). These eighteenth-century observations describe aspects of what we now refer to as secondary trauma.

According to Levenson and Ruef (1992), researchers have failed to agree upon a single definition of empathy and report that this term can refer to three different phenomena: (a) knowing what another person is feeling, (b) feeling what another person is feeling (and this is particularly germane to understanding secondary trauma and perhaps the notion of sympathy), and (c) responding compassionately.

© The Author(s), under exclusive license to Springer Nature Switzerland AG 2023

R. W. Motta, *Secondary Trauma*, https://doi.org/10.1007/978-3-031-44308-4_1

Therefore, secondary traumatization is best seen as knowing and feeling the distress of another person and responding compassionately to help the sufferer and relieve their distress.

**When Does Empathy Develop?** This capability to react to the emotions of others appears to develop early in one's life. Cummings et al. (1981) demonstrated that children, even those less than 1 year of age, are not only aware of family members' expressions of anger and affection but appear to have an emotional reaction to them. Expressions of anger in adults appeared to act as stressors and caused distress in young children. Similarly, affectionate interactions between child caretakers were most often responded to by overt signs of pleasure on the part of the children. From this we might surmise that the ability to connect with another's emotions is not necessarily taught but seems to be a built-in response that is displayed by children younger than 1 year of age.

In a twin study of the genetic and environmental contributions to empathy (Knafo et al., 2008), it was reported that empathy encompasses both cognitive and affective aspects and it is the latter that might be referred to as a vicarious emotional response (Hoffman, 1988). The cognitive aspect entails a recognition or comprehension that, for example, another is in distress. In terms of our discussion of secondary traumatization, the affective, or vicarious emotional aspect of empathy, refers to the sense of distress experienced by the observer of another who is in distress. Vicarious affective responding appears to be stable and to show both genetic and environmental components. The contribution of environmental influences appears to be more prominent when vicarious emotional responding activates prosocial responding. Stated another way, while empathy relies upon a significant genetic or inborn contribution, prosocial behavior appears as a learned response that is acquired by very young children (Hoffman, 1988).

**Ancestral Underpinnings of Secondary Trauma** While it may be gratifying and ego-enhancing to believe that the capacity for empathy is a uniquely human characteristic, it is not. In 1964 Masserman et al. trained rhesus monkeys to associate bar pressing with causing shock to be delivered to a monkey in an adjoining cage. These researchers offered a food reward if the monkeys in the first cage would intentionally give a shock to a monkey in a second cage. These researchers discovered that most monkeys trained to deliver the shock for a food reward would not do so and were willing to suffer hunger if eating meant delivering pain to another monkey. One monkey reportedly went 12 days without food to avoid inflicting harm to the monkey in the adjoining cage.

Miller et al. (1963) trained monkeys to avoid shock by bar pressing. When these monkeys viewed another monkey being shocked nearby, they began bar pressing even though they were experiencing no shock themselves. In this we see primate compassionate prosocial responding. The monkeys also bar pressed when watching a soundless video of a monkey in distress and fear and even bar pressed when shown a photograph of a monkey in pain. Studies such as these provide compelling data to support the position that we humans, and other mammals, may be "hardwired" for empathy-based phenomena like secondary traumatization. We may like to believe that compassionate responding is a noble and uniquely human characteristic, but the data suggest otherwise.

Hrdy (2011) suggests that one of the origins of our emotional connection with others may have been linked to cooperative childcare practices of our ape ancestors who lived a few million years ago. Cooperative childcare involves entrusting the raising of offspring to others so that there is a sharing of childcare and more efficient use of resources. In times of limited food availability and the need for group hunting, cooperative childcare became a more effective tool for promoting group survival than noncooperative practices. This form of cooperation facilitates and necessitates trust in and knowing of others. An ancestral ape must be able to ascertain the intentions and goodwill of another to entrust the caring of their offspring to others. And, because the recognition of the intentions of others offered a survival advantage over not being able to do so, it was passed down to future generations.

From the above we can see that "mind reading," or perhaps intention reading, may have grown out of the need for cooperative offspring caring, and such caring was based on a need to survive when resources were limited. This form of offspring cooperative rearing is said to date back to the Pleistocene era or Ice Age. Exclusive childcare, where one rears their own offspring, appears to be a far less stressful way to rear ape offspring in comparison to cooperative rearing as infanticide by male and female chimpanzees and gorillas is a leading cause of death. So, entrusting the care of one's infant to others requires a leap of faith in the other's positive intentions. The evolutionary advantage of cooperative childcare and being able to "read" others assured that these capabilities would be carried into future generations. Hrdy claims that the development of cooperative childcare in apes was a critical point in later human evolution. And while the overall impact of cooperative childrearing was advantageous in an evolutionary sense, it may also have been the seed that spawned empathy, compassion, emotional contagion, and when life became problematic, secondary traumatization. One must be able to read and connect with others if one is to become emotionally upset by the distress of others.

From the above it would appear that the ability to connect with and understand the mindset or emotionality of others may have conferred an evolutionary advantage and that we humans may be "hardwired" or genetically programmed for empathic awareness and understanding. These wiring speculations blossomed into active research programs because of the serendipitous observations of a group of Italian researchers.

**Neurophysiological Underpinnings** In 1992, the neurophysiologist Giacomo Rizzolatti and his research team at the University of Parma were investigating how the brain coordinates the various muscles involved in hand movements. They did this by inserting electrodes in the frontal cortex of macaque monkeys and monitoring neural activity. On returning to the lab to have lunch, they accidentally discovered that monkey neurons fired when they observed the experimenters eating, and these were the same neurons that fired when they, the monkeys, brought food to their mouths (Rizzolatti, & Fadiga, 1999). These observations led to a highly active field of research on "mirror neurons." While almost all this research has been done with monkeys, it has also been conducted with rodents and birds. The discovery of mirror neurons and their potential role in cooperative behavior, development of culture, and autism led to a flurry of research activities. It is easy to speculate that what we call secondary trauma may likely be "hardwired" at a basic neuronal level, and this wiring may have taken place because of the evolutionary advantage noted above. Using this line of thinking, secondary traumatization may be seen as having neurophysiological underpinnings related to mirror neurons.

Much of the early excitement over the role of mirror neurons in the development of social behaviors and in emotional connectedness has waned following skepticism over their essential nature (e.g., Hickok, 2009). For example, even though macaques were initially studied, it has been noted that much of the learning of these monkeys does not come through imitation, and therefore mirroring explains little of their behavior. Similarly, research with humans has been difficult to conduct, and this research has suggested a limited explanatory utility of mirror neurons in understanding social awareness and autism and in learning processes. Despite these inconclusive findings, the research on mirror neurons has pointed to the possibility that specific brain areas may play a role in our ability to understand, learn from, and connect with others. Nevertheless, difficulty in identifying specific brain areas has had a dampening effect on mirror neuron research.

**Summary Comments on Origins of Secondary Trauma** We know that secondary traumatization is real and that it represents a spread or contagion of distress from one to another. If it were a virus, we would have to conclude that it is a highly contagious one. But why do we carry this burdensome capacity? From the reviewed material, the capability to be impacted by the emotional state of others afforded human beings a group evolutionary survival advantage, and as a result the capacity to develop secondary trauma may be an inherited characteristic. Sensitivity to and responsiveness to the feelings and distress of others have been noted over the lifespan and appear to be present in children before their first birthday. Further, this capability is not limited to human beings. It seems to be shown in primates that will go to significant lengths to prevent their brethren from encountering harm and distress. For such caring behavior to occur, the monkeys must be aware on some level of the potential distress in other monkeys. Neurophysiological studies have revealed neuronal underpinnings for being able to pick up on the behavior of others or even their intentions. In all, the available research observations appear to show that our ability to be sensitive and reactive to the emotions and distress of others is at least partially inborn just as are many other human characteristics that have been of value in our evolutionary history.

# Chapter 2
# Childhood Secondary Trauma

The capability of experiencing secondary trauma reactions begins at a young age and is not an exclusive capacity of humans as shown in Chap. 1. Regardless of age of development, secondary traumatic stress disorder (STSD) has several similarities to posttraumatic stress disorder (PTSD) with the primary differences being the source of the distress and the magnitude of the subsequent emotional disruption. For PTSD the distressing event is experienced directly, but in STSD the source is indirect in that it is an emotional response to another's difficulties. Although there is no unanimity of opinion, the consequences of PTSD appear, in general, to be more debilitating than those of secondary traumatization (e.g., Suozzi & Motta, 2004). For example, among mental health therapists who treat clients with diverse demographic backgrounds and who might expect to experience secondary trauma, there is a low rate of PTSD symptoms of 0–4% (e.g., Adams et al., 2001; Jenkins & Baird, 2002; Wasco & Campbell, 2002). These differences between PTSD and secondary trauma will be highlighted in later sections of this book, but try as one might, a set of diagnostic criteria for STSD will not be found in any official source from organizations such as the American Psychological Association or American Psychiatric Association. While there is no diagnostic classification for STSD or secondary trauma in the *Diagnostic and Statistical Manual (DSM)* of the American Psychiatric Association, this is not the case with PTSD as it was first included in its third edition (third ed. [*DSM III*]; American Psychiatric Association, 1980) where it was listed under anxiety disorders. PTSD is now listed in the *DSM-5* under "Trauma and Stress-Related Disorders" (p. 265) (5th ed. [*DSM-5*]; American Psychiatric Association, 2013), but it is clear to practicing clinicians that, regardless of the *DSM* edition, anxiety and depression are central components of the distress of PTSD and this might also be said of STSD.

One source of this anxiety in STSD is often a response to a perceived loss of the environment to which one had become accustomed and the difficulty accepting and adapting to these newfound changes. This response to perceived loss is especially pronounced in children. This chapter will cover several prototypical examples of childhood secondary trauma and address some of the major causes of and interventions for this disorder.

© The Author(s), under exclusive license to Springer Nature Switzerland AG 2023

R. W. Motta, *Secondary Trauma*, https://doi.org/10.1007/978-3-031-44308-4_2

## 2.1 Overview of Contributors to Secondary Trauma in Children: The Role of Loss

If one were to examine the various sources of secondary trauma among children, one might see that anxiety, often accompanied by depression, plays a central role in response to many types of perceived loss. The loss could be that of the security the child once felt and that is now unavailable due to one or both parents and other caretakers being confronted with an all-consuming stressor. The parental or caretaker stress could be due to events such as emotional difficulties, financial losses, natural disasters, loss of a bond between partners, separation due to incarceration, medical problems, drug addiction, detention following illegal immigration, or any number of other stressful events. These events, whatever their nature, typically cause a disruption from what the child had been accustomed to as compared to what is now taking place (Motta, 2005). Perhaps the child has lost his or her secure role as a dependent who needs attention and now has been thrust into the role of the caretaker to overwhelmed parents. The child's perceptions of loss might also be due to a current lack of emotional support and nurturance. Children in these situations note that their caretakers or family members have changed and now seem less available than they were previously. The present is no longer what it used to be. For example, the parent who has developed a drug addiction, or is now consumed with the pain of a medical problem, or is going through a divorce is no longer emotionally or physically available to the child as they had been in the past (e.g., Lombardo, 2007). Similarly, a sibling with whom a child had a close relationship is now ill and suffering or is emotionally troubled and preoccupied and in need of support. The child is now deeply concerned with the sibling's suffering and is also troubled by the disruption of the predictability of their former relationship

All these scenarios present themselves as a change from the way things were and a loss of support. They have a destabilizing and distressing impact. These events may be perceived as personally felt disruptions to the secondarily traumatized child. They represent an unwelcome change from the way things used to be. The loss of formerly available support and emotional nurturance can evoke apprehension, distress, and depression on the part of the child. While children are typically playful and show curiosity in their environments, the child experiencing secondary trauma symptoms will often come across as sullen, moody, withdrawn, and on edge. Let us look at two of a multitude of possible case examples.

## 2.2 Marty's Response to the Sex Change of His Father

Although Marty was a typically developing 8-year-old boy who was doing well academically and had a group of friends both in and out of school, a change was taking place in his life. His grades began to slide, and he was becoming increasingly isolated and sullen. He was referred to counseling after a suicide attempt in which he tried to cut his wrists with a razor. Suicide attempts at this age are highly unusual. The Centers for

Disease Control (2014) and Anderson et al. (2016) suggest that the rate of suicide in this age group is fewer than two in one million. It turns out that what was taking place in Marty's life was that his father was in the process of becoming a woman. The father was so preoccupied with his sexual and gender identity concerns and so troubled by this upcoming major life change that he had little time for his son, a son with whom he once had a close and loving relationship. The father had also pulled away from Marty's mother. The combined impact of his dad's self-absorption and his mom's consuming distress over where she fit within this evolving situation left Marty with feelings of being emotionally abandoned, unwanted, and unable to help his distressed parents despite his desire to do so. He sensed that his mom and dad were both unhappy and self-absorbed and his prevailing feeling was one of emotional abandonment. Marty felt that he was once part of a family and now he was adrift and had to fend for himself. The anxiety and depression and feelings of both helplessness and hopelessness that circumstances were unlikely to change are what prompted his suicide attempt.

Marty saw himself pushed into the role of a caregiver, not a care receiver, and as a result experienced significant distress. He tried whatever he knew, which was very little, to help his parents with their perceived distress. He was confused and could do little other than repeatedly ask his parents if they were OK. He was alone and adrift. His world had radically changed, and he had few tools to manage his situation. His utter despair drove him to the extreme act of attempting to end his life.

This was a complex case that eventuated in family therapy where the emphasis was on an expression of feelings and a recognition of the feelings of others. Although Marty's father went ahead with his change of identity, he stayed with his wife, and they maintained a loving though nonsexual bond. Therapy helped them to become more aware of Marty's plight and allowed them to understand their own and their partner's feelings. As a result of family intervention, Marty improved rapidly and made a good adjustment overall. This positive outcome for him appeared to be due to the expression and recognition of his feelings and of those feelings being attended to by his parents. What one sees here is a child secondarily traumatized by the distress of his parents and his evolving feelings of aloneness and abandonment. Once Marty's parents were able to clearly see the distress their child was experiencing and were able to provide him with understanding and emotional support, his situation changed radically. Marty's case provides us with a common theme often seen in cases of childhood secondary traumatization, that is, being burdened with the problems of others, losing emotional support and comfort from loving caretakers, and as a result feeling frightened, sullen, alone, and abandoned.

Let us look at another case of childhood secondary trauma.

## 2.3 Juan's Family Decides to Migrate to the USA

There appears to be a fundamental human desire to migrate and find a better life for one's family (Daniels, 2002). This drive is what was behind Juan's undocumented parents' unsuccessful effort to find residence in the USA. Regrettably, to stem immigration across the Mexican border, the then attorney general, Jeff Sessions, announced a "zero tolerance" policy in May 2018. What this policy did was to jail and then deport undocumented immigrants and to separate them from their children, the latter of whom were placed in "shelters." The vitriolic protests and outrage that this policy produced resulted in then-president Donald Trump signing an executive order to end family separation and supplant it with family detention. So now parents and their children were treated as criminals and were all detained and then deported. The former policy of separation placed children in dreary shelters, which were little more than child prisons, and many of them were later transferred to foster care. Although the family detention plan now addressed the separation from children problem, efforts to reunite those separated children often failed, and to this day many have not found their parents (Domomoske & Gonzalez, 2018).

Juan, age 10, his sister, age eight, and their two parents were jailed in their attempt to cross the US-Mexican border. This close-knit and loving family was now being treated like a group of common criminals and placed in what amounted to little more than a cage. Their alienation from the small community from which they came, where everyone knew each other for many years and where the community functioned as an extended family, was a culture shock of horrific proportions. Juan was traumatized not only by his own fear but also by the terrible distress that he saw his father, mother, and sister enduring. His mom and dad from whom he formerly sought comfort were tormented with anxiety and were somber, fretful, and chronically distressed. Whereas adults are often able to put things in perspective and see that their current circumstances are likely to change, children simply lack this facility owing to their limited life experiences. To Juan, what was taking place was a tragedy that produced extreme levels of anxiety and seemed to have no end. In the past he was able to look to his mother and father for support, guidance, and discipline. Now he saw them as often tearful, trembling in fear, and as enduring harsh treatment and alien surroundings. They did not have much reserve left over to provide needed support for their children. Jail was simply not the place to be for this young child, even though his parents and sister were with him.

It is often the case that children are more impacted by the reactions of their parents who are facing a traumatic stressor than by the stressor itself (e.g., Freud & Burlingham, 1942). This was certainly the case with Juan. He was far more troubled by the fact that his family members were all extremely distressed and overwhelmed than he was by sleeping in a crowded and strange jail cell.

This vulnerability to the reaction of family members has been noted in early literature. Freud and Burlingham (1942) found that the degree of distress in response to parental reactions to the bombing of London in World War II exceeded the fear of the bombing itself. Ziv and Israeli (1973) noted that the bombardment of kibbutzim in Israel troubled children less than the extent to which their parents were terrorized by the bombing. A similar situation where children are more impacted by their family's reactions than by the traumatic event itself was seen with Hurricane Sandy, which hit the eastern coast of the USA in October of 2012. Children who were rescued from their now-inundated homes appeared to be far more upset by the emotional distress of their parents who had to flee their surroundings than by the rising water levels and floating debris in their homes (Motta, 2021). This greater impact of the emotional state of caretakers than of actual potentially traumatizing events may be due to children not understanding the monumental demands involved in either rebuilding their homes or finding a new home, or the real potential for disaster in a bombing, but they are fully aware of the immediate distress and upset of their parents and their own resulting insecurity. Parents are seen as protectors and as providers of the foundation that makes life predictable. When the parents are viewed as being overwhelmed, this produces extreme levels of fear in the children, more so than the actual loss of their toys and personal belongings and separation from friends and acquaintances.

Although his parents were devastated when they were sent back to Mexico, Juan was relieved. Things did not turn out the way his mother and father may have hoped, but for Juan it was a tremendous relief to no longer see them in the extreme distress that they experienced when they were imprisoned. The family was now back in the familiar and supportive community where they previously lived. Like what took place during Hurricane Sandy and similar situations that produced overwhelming stress on caretakers, Juan had responded more to his parents' reactions than any personal discomfort of his own.

Distressing as Juan's situation was, it could have been worse. Had he been separated from his jailed parents, he likely would have suffered behavioral problems, developmental delays, extreme separation anxiety, ambivalent feeling toward his parents whom he may have been seen as blameworthy for allowing this separation to occur, aggression toward his parents, depression, appetite problems, and intense shame over having witnessed the arrest of his parents. The traumatic impact of family separation can also have lifelong consequences including difficulty forming relationships, distrust, and profound feelings of low self-worth (Yoshikawa & Kalil, 2011). So, in this case, detention with Juan's family was more desirable than having been wrenched from them as had taken place in the former US family separation plan.

## 2.4 Secondary Trauma in Children Under the Age of 5

Children under the age of 5 are so entirely dependent upon caretakers that the disruption of this dependency bond can have profound consequences. The response of very young children to the distress and emotional unavailability of caretakers is similar to their response to an actual loss such as might occur due to caretaker death, incarceration, abandonment, or severe impairment. Regardless of whether the parent is physically or emotionally unavailable, the response on the child's part appears to be one of despair. My parent is lost and therefore I am lost (Whitten, 2008). The very young child's despair is not the classic emotional contagion seen in secondary traumatization but rather is an extreme distress of abandonment borne out of emotional unavailability of caretakers (Bowlby, 1968/1982). Emotional stability and physiological balance are inextricably tied to the physical and emotional presence of the caretaker. This stability is essential in very young children who are utterly helpless to fend for themselves. When the caretaker is physically or emotionally not present, the young child suffers in the extreme.

Bowlby (1968/1982), following an extensive investigation of separation from the primary caregiver, concluded that there were a series of stages that the abandoned young child passes through and that this sequence is independent of the child's exact age, background, health status, time length of separation, and other factors. These stages are protest, despair, and detachment. The first stage of protest involves agitation where the child might frantically search for the caregiver they once had. They may throw themselves around or excitedly orient to any sound or other stimulus that reminds the child of the lost caretaking figure. The next stage, despair, entails a disinterest in and detachment from the environment. It may be seen in the expression of a low energy level, withdrawal, and lack of interest in any form of activity. In the final stage of detachment, the child no longer responds to attachment figures and will appear as remote, aloof, and unavailable. This is not a simple forgetting but rather a predictable defensive reaction to the pain or loss and the building of a wall against the experience of further pain. Again, the issue is not just the physical absence of the caretaker that matters because in many instances even substitute caretakers will be incapable of breaking through the young child's detachment. What is lost to the child is the emotional presence and provision of nurturance from the caretaker. This form of loss blurs the boundaries between primary and secondary trauma, but the fact that the traumatic experience entails a loss of emotional support and nurturance from another human could arguably be viewed as an example of secondary trauma.

## 2.5 Specific Sources of Secondary Trauma in Children Older Than Age 5

There are multiple sources of secondary trauma and loss in school-age children. There are losses due to serious illness leading to death, to suicide, or to homicide and many others. If the loss is due to the death of a family member, the child confronts an unwelcome realization that death is both real and permanent. Complicating matters further not only does the child mourn the loss of family members but can also mourn for the mourners (Worden, 1991), and this is the essence of secondary trauma: distress over another's distress. Confusion and further distress can be added to the emotional upset that a child feels over the loss of a loved one when the child's caretaker or parent and other significant people in the child's life fail to address the glaring loss. This failure to deal with the painful loss of a family member by adults in the child's life may be due to the latter's own difficulty in dealing with their feelings over a death and attempts to shield a child from the pain of the loss. "It isn't unusual for the most caring parent in the world to forget a child's birthday because of grief, and children don't know how to make their needs known or to articulate loss. They often lack the words to put to their emotions and since their lives are just beginning, how can we expect them to understand life's endings?" (Kubler-Ross & Kessler, 2014, p. 160). School-age children, whether classmates or not, who witness other students suffer over a family loss can develop their own secondary trauma reactions. Terr (1981), for example, described these secondary trauma reactions in the case of the contagious nature of childhood traumatic experiences of nonfamily member age-mates that came about because of a kidnap attempt involving an entire school bus. Children who became aware of the suffering of those youngsters who were kidnapped suffered along with them.

## 2.6 Intentional Taking of Life

Homicide or suicide within a family presents even greater challenges to youth than do deaths from natural or accidental causes. In the child's mind, the former losses don't fit within the normal context of their understanding of life and living. Upper elementary school-age children and beyond begin to recognize the fragility and vulnerability of life when a homicide or suicide takes place. While the primary survivors, that is, those closest to the now deceased, may experience PTSD reactions, secondary trauma can extend to larger school populations who are now struck with the hard-to-fathom intentional taking of life. The normal belief in the continuity of life is now supplanted by feelings of vulnerability, threat, and doubt (Steele, 1992). Again, the issue of loss comes to the fore. Previous perceptions of invulnerability and the unquestioning acceptance of a life that is not threatened by wholly unexpected causes are now supplanted by perceptions of vulnerability and apprehension. The emotional upheaval that intentional loss of life precipitates appears to spread to other children in an almost contagious-like fashion (Hatfield et al., 1994).

## 2.7 War and Secondary Trauma

Children whose parents have been involved in war situations can often acquire secondary trauma reactions in response to their parents' distress over combat and noncombat experiences. One of the original systematic studies in this area was that of Rosenheck and Nathan (1985) who found that children essentially acquired their parents' imagery and fears related to the Vietnam War and tended to reenact these experiences in fantasy. Rosenheck (1986) noted that children of veterans who were overly close with their fathers tended to carry the father's emotional burdens into their adult lives, and these burdens influenced their own choice of careers, lifestyle, and choice of partner.

Williams and Williams (1987) found that the children of veterans suffered from depression, emotional distancing, and behavioral and school-related problems. Suozzi and Motta (2004) showed that a father's combat exposure led to PTSD-like symptoms in the children of Vietnam veterans suffering from PTSD compared to those veterans without PTSD. In fact, children showed response delays to color naming Vietnam combat-related words on a modified Stroop procedure, an objective response time measure designed to assess secondary trauma in this study. The Stroop procedure used here was a variant of the original method in which color naming reaction times are recorded in response to color words printed in congruent and incongruent colors (Stroop, 1935). For example, it takes a person longer to name the ink color of the word *red* when the word is printed in green ink than when it is printed in the congruent color of red. In the Suozzi and Motta (2004) study, Vietnam-relevant words, such as Nam, Cong, and Medivac and so on took longer to color name when the children's fathers had Vietnam-related PTSD than when they did not. This study provided an objective way of measuring the presence of secondary traumatization. The hypervigilance and startle reactions shown by PTSD-positive veterans appear to impact their children in such a way that they too begin showing these reactions. This form of emotional contagion, or secondary traumatization, is common in the children of war veterans. Again, what we see here is a strong contagious-like reaction on the part of offspring to their parent's distress. This distress in response to parental reactions, as previously shown (Freud & Burlingham, 1942; Motta, 2021; Ziv & Israeli, 1973), can have a greater impact on children than the actual situation that produced the danger.

## 2.8 Natural Disaster

In general, trauma and secondary trauma that have their origins in natural disasters, such as floods, earthquakes, and hurricanes are less impactful than those resulting from personal assaults, such as rapes; emotional, physical, and sexual abuse; and muggings (e.g., Boscarino et al., 2006; Motta, 2020). Remission rates for natural disasters, 60%, are also higher than what one might see from having experienced personal illness, which is about 30% (e.g., Morina et al., 2014). Morina et al. suggest that the reason personal illness has a low remission rate is that the individual carries the potential traumatic experience around with them. Personal attacks of various kinds have remission rates between these two. From this we can see traumatic experiences and the consequent secondary trauma that impact those connected to the trauma victim are influenced by several factors including type of trauma, age, gender (females are more at risk), socioeconomic status, premorbid adjustment, social support, perceived duration, and intensity of the trauma and perhaps several other factors (Motta, 2020).

Regarding secondary trauma in children, the major reason why specific types of trauma matter more than others is that they might have a differential impact on the primarily traumatized person. The intensity of response of the traumatized person then affects the magnitude of response in the secondarily traumatized child. As is true with primary trauma and PTSD, it is likely that young female children of lower socioeconomic status, who lack social support and whose prior emotional adjustment may have been poorer, are likely to be those who are most vulnerable to developing secondary trauma. However, regardless of demographic characteristics, the intensity of the distress response of the person who experienced primary trauma and to whom the child had a close relationship is a major factor in the development of secondary trauma in the child. If there is a close child-caretaker bond and the traumatized individual is impacted in a significant and enduring way, then the child is at high risk for developing secondary trauma responses. Let us examine a case example.

## 2.9 Dora and Hurricane Sandy

Hurricane Sandy hit the East Coast of the USA in 2012. Although it was not a major hurricane in terms of sustained wind speeds, its timing resulted in a good deal of devastation. On Long Island, New York, where 13-year-old Dora and her single mother, Jean, lived, the storm hit during a high tide. The combination of tides and winds was devastating. It was somewhat unexpected that Dora, who had been struggling with both learning, anxiety, and social problems, did not appear to be particularly upset in seeing the rising tides, unmoored boats floating down the street, and howling winds. Unfortunately, the same could not be said about her mother, Jean.

In the beginning of the hurricane, Jean put on a brave face and seemed to know instinctively that it was important to show her daughter that all would turn out well and that there was no need to panic. It may be that this explains why Dora was not overly fearful at first. However, as the water level began to rise in the home, Jean became overwhelmed and subsequently began shrieking from the windows and loudly begging for help from the police and fire departments on the telephone. It was at this point that Dora, seeing her mother becoming unglued, panicked, and started screaming and crying. Eventually, a large police van was able to get to the house and bring Dora and Jean to a public shelter in one of the local high schools. Once securely away from the flood waters, Jean began to gain control of herself, but Dora continued to be panicked and inconsolable. She developed intermittent panic attacks that went on for 6 months and refused to leave her mother's side.

A social worker was assigned to this family and held weekly sessions with Dora and Jean. Dora's panic attacks grew less frequent, and over a period of months, she began to return to her former self. It was the social worker's opinion that what threw Dora into a frenzied state was the image and memories of her mother frantically yelling and calling out for help. Dora's only perceived support had collapsed, and Dora collapsed along with it. Ultimately, Jean's reattainment of stability allowed Dora to bring her own anxieties under control. In the early phase of the storm, Dora displayed curiosity but no excessive fear. It was the witnessing of her mother, her sole support, becoming overwhelmed that caused Dora to also become frantic. Again, we see that the traumatic experience, although potentially difficult to endure, appears to have less of a negative impact than the response of the caregiver. Added negative contributors to Dora's panicked responding were her gender, the fact that she was young, that she had specific adjustment challenges before Sandy, and that she and her single mom led a somewhat isolated existence that was relatively lacking in social support. It is likely that if she were older, had a good adjustment, and had greater social support, her reaction would not have been so extreme.

The case of Dora highlights the fact that there are many factors that influence the possible development of secondary trauma reactions in children and that a major one is the reaction of the caregiver. Dora lost the security and support of her mother when the latter was overwhelmed by a natural disaster. As a result, Dora also became overcome by anxiety and an inability to cope. When Dora regained her mom's reassuring presence, she regained her emotional footing.

## 2.10 Children Who Are Secondarily Traumatized by the Childhood Trauma of Their Parents

One often hears the reputed biblical expression that the sins of the father are passed onto the son. There is an essential truth in this expression that is applicable to secondary traumatization. In general, children who have been abused, or exposed to other extreme traumatic experiences, often pass on the emotional consequence of these traumas to their children once they have grown up. The victimization of a child tends to eventually result in the victimization of their own children when they become adults (Figley, 1989).

As a rule, most forms of intense traumatic experience, including that of long-running child abuse, result in some form of diminution and negative sense of self and distrust of the environment (Motta, 2020, p. 19). These negative sequelae can then be passed on to offspring. Regardless of whether the trauma is due to torture, sexual, emotional, or physical abuse or a combination of these, the recipient of this abuse often develops a low and loathsome sense of self. In being abused, a child may be treated as an object as in sexual abuse or as an unworthy and deficient individual as might occur in cases of physical and emotional abuse. These early self-views are formed because the child interprets their caretaker's abusive behavior as an indication of their own lack of value. If you are beaten, tortured, sexually assaulted, or the recipient of continued demeaning evaluations, of what value are you? Your self-perception is one of valuelessness. You are a flawed and deficient being. Your lack of self-worth and accompanying anger and anxiety over having been maltreated often results in an inability to regulate your own emotions (Osborne et al., 2021).

So, then what happens when the person who harbors deep insecurities, emotional pain, and pervasive self-doubts has a child? After all, their child is a product of them. How could such a deficient being as themselves produce a child who is inherently valuable and in possession of characteristics that would warrant unconditional love, nurturance, and approval? The answer to this question is that it is highly unlikely that the child of an abused or otherwise traumatized parent will receive unconditional approval, love, and support. The children of traumatized parents are secondarily traumatized. "Children of parents with a history of trauma, particularly trauma that is severe in nature (e.g., exposure to atrocities, repeated sexual abuse, torture), exhibit a variety of secondary symptoms that may recapitulate the PTSD of the parent" (Williams, 1998, p. 98). The parent is wary, distrusting, and emotionally dysregulated and has a deficient sense of self following a history of severe trauma or abuse. This parent or caretaker, who views themselves as deeply flawed, interprets their child's typical behavior as problematic, negative, and a reminder of their own deficiencies. The child of a traumatized parent is distressed not only by their own undeserved maltreatment but is often burdened by viewing their caretaker as irritable, troubled, and given to angry outbursts. The offspring of the traumatized parent, from the beginnings of their awareness, see themselves as unlovable, deficient, and flawed and come to deeply distrust the punitive environment in which they find themselves. Trauma, in this scenario, has been transferred intergenerationally from parent to child.

## 2.11 Intergenerational Trauma Transmission: The Case of Victor

The intergenerational transmission of trauma as a form of secondary traumatization can take several different forms such as those that are related to war experiences of parents, to being impacted by parents who had been abused as children, or even to the passing on of traumatic experiences due to events such as the Holocaust. In the Holocaust, some adult children who did not have the same terrible experience as their parents can nevertheless be impacted and encounter elevations of anxiety, depression, vulnerability, and lack of trust, although others seem to cope well and do not show these symptoms (e.g., Danieli 1998; Kassai & Motta, 2006; van IJzendoorn et al., 2003). Some studies have examined the transfer of Holocaust-related trauma to the third-generation grandchildren and have found that the negative effects appear to dissipate with the passage of time (Kassai & Motta, 2006; Perlstein & Motta, 2012). Mental health counselors are particularly aware of the intergenerational impact of trauma within families and regularly treat such problems. A typical case of trauma transferred within a family is seen in the case of Victor.

Victor came into therapy as a comparatively successful guidance counselor. He indicated that he was seeking therapy because of an inability to form emotional attachments. He was now in his 50s and reported a history of failed relationships. An examination of his history revealed that his grandparents on both his mother's and father's side had abused Victor's parents. On his mother's side, there were reports of sexual abuse by her father and alcoholism on the part of the mother, Victor's grandmother. On his father's side, there was emotional and physical abuse by both of Victor's grandparents and subsequent placement of his father in unstable and abusive foster care settings. With these backgrounds of his parents, it would be highly unlikely for them to be ready for effective parenting, and they were not. Victor remembers his father beating him and verbally abusing him and referring to him as "the shit head" because of his problems at school. His mother was simultaneously sexually provocative, emotionally unavailable, and physically abusive. Victor painfully recalls at the age of 10 being invited into his parents' bed where his mother, scantily attired, would "spoon" with him. This caused extreme anxiety for Victor. It did not help that his father responded to his son's presence in bed with irritability and hostility. One of his most painful memories is when his mother sent him into the basement and then followed him downstairs and locked the door behind her. He was 8 years old at the time and it appears that he had engaged in some minor transgression that he can no longer recall. His mother began hitting him with a 2 × 4 piece of lumber. He reports that he felt he was going to be killed by his mother's efforts to hit him in the head. When asked why his mother could be so dangerously abusive, he states that he believes that she was having a psychotic episode at the time because he could not recall what provoked the attack. The intense memories of his fear of death at the hands of his own mother have indelibly etched themselves on his now adult mind.

Victor describes his childhood as a nightmare where he was abused both at home and at school. He did poorly academically and was bullied by the other children. Despite his poor academic and equally poor social functioning, he eventually was able to do well in college and obtain a graduate degree in guidance counseling. He stated that he chose this profession to spare the children under his purview the agonizing upbringing that he endured.

When he entered college, Victor availed himself of the services of the college counseling center and stayed in counseling for 4 years. His stated reasons for seeking counseling were anxiety, self-doubt, occasional explosive outbursts, and failed relationships. He sought therapy over the subsequent years and reported that he had been receiving counseling and therapy with an array of therapists for over 30 years. Now being treated by a trauma specialist, he is finally able to see that his self-doubts, distrust, and a myriad of relationship problems were not due to his own deficiencies but rather to the fact that he was the recipient of ongoing childhood abuse. This abuse caused both a negative sense of self and a distrust of relationships. As a result of insights gained in therapy, especially the knowledge of the intergenerational transmission of trauma, he slowly began to develop the ability to value himself and to see that there was nothing inherently deficient about him and that he currently responds as most children would who are brought up in abusive environments. In summary, Victor has begun to accept and appreciate himself and to recognize his inherent self-worth. Interpersonal relationships continue to be a problem in that he has difficulty with emotional commitments. And yet Victor is optimistic that he is making progress in overcoming the hurdle of an abusive childhood. He is fully aware of the intergenerational nature of his abuse and is moving in a constructive and hopeful direction. When asked what he sees as the reason for his progress, he states that he is now able to accept himself as a person who has relationship problems due to abusive parenting rather than seeing himself as a person hiding numerous deficiencies.

## 2.12 Media Impact: Anita's Fears

Children are capable of being secondarily traumatized by what they see and hear in various forms of media (e.g., Schlenger et al., 2002). Again, what unnerves them most, just as in natural disasters as described above, appears to be the reaction of the caretaker adults in their lives. However, they can also become troubled by the sights and sounds of other people suffering, by the concern shown by media commentators, and by the actual events being graphically and theatrically depicted.

Anita, a 7-year-old, was such a child. Anita and her parents were glued to the television amid reports of Saddam Hussein's Iraqi military launching Scud missiles toward Israel. The media depicted this as the "Scud missile crisis." She and her parents were unnerved by the TV coverage of the missiles' explosive impacts and by the subsequent engagement of the USA against Iraq in 2003. Anita's specifically stated fear was that the Scud missiles would land on her home in Long Island, New York.

The range of variants of the mobile Scud missile is approximately 100 to 400 miles. It is a tactical weapon used in local conflicts. It is incapable of reaching the USA from Iraq. Even though Anita was informed of this, it did not seem to ameliorate her anxieties. What she was reacting to was the concern and emotional impact shown by her parents, by the cries of those on the receiving end of this weapon, and by the media hyping the danger in order to boost news show ratings. The technical information about missile range was lost on her as it would be on any child of her age. Anita was experiencing a strong anxiety reaction primarily because those around her and on the TV were displaying fear and concern. Her once secure and safe environment was now seen as threatened, and she reacted accordingly. "The level of threat experienced by primary survivors impacts their (the child's) reaction …" (Williams, 1998, p. 99). The unique aspect of the case described here was that Anita was secondarily traumatized by parents who were also secondarily traumatized. The parents reacted with fear and distress to what they were viewing on television. Anita then reacted to the concern that she saw in her parents in addition to the actual depictions of suffering from those being rocketed. By creating fear in parents and other caregivers, the media has been responsible for a great deal of the secondary traumatization of children.

It should be of little surprise that Anita seemed to not be consoled by her parents informing her that Scud missiles were incapable of reaching their Long Island home. Children are generally unresponsive to such technical information. They are reacting to the potential disruption of their security owing to their caretakers' distress. This should be of no surprise as adults are also frequently unconvinced by technical details. Consider the person who has a flying phobia. Informing such fearful people that airline travel is the safest mode of transportation on a mile-to-mile or hour-to-hour basis in comparison to any other form of transportation will often not alleviate their dread of walking down the jetway toward the waiting airliner. Their fear and that of secondarily traumatized children are not based on technical data. They are based on perceived disruptions and threats to one's safety.

What ultimately helped Anita was a therapist informing her parents that she was reacting to their fears. They decided to stop exposing their child to fear-inducing TV programs and commentary and stayed away from watching these disruptive sources themselves. Anita was assured that there was no longer any danger, but what helped her overcome her fears was her perception that her parents were no longer unnerved. Anita regained the sense of safety and security that she once had, and as a result her apprehensions began to subside.

## 2.13 Secondary Trauma Treatment Strategies for Children

While the focus of this book is on secondary trauma involving family members, health-care professionals, and first responders, some comments are warranted regarding interventions for children. Although not always the case, children do not generally require traditional one-on-one psychotherapy to deal with secondary trauma. Rather what is needed is that the child should experience a normalization or reestablishment of the way things used to be to overcome their perceptions of loss of their familiar environments and expectations. The cases presented above show, for example, that Marty's anxieties over the loss of the dad he knew were alleviated when it was shown that his dad was still there for him. Juan's anxieties over witnessing the distress of his parents abated when his family was returned to its familiar environment. Dora's reaction to Hurricane Sandy was a reaction to her mother's fears and not the hurricane itself. Victor was exposed to intergenerational trauma, and leaving his abusive household had salutary effects on him. The counseling he received did help him, but it appeared that separating himself from the negative influence of his family was most helpful. And finally, Anita overcame her fears when she viewed her parents as being in control and not being troubled by the televised Scud missile attacks.

The secondary traumas that children encounter, like secondary trauma itself, can arise from numerous sources, but because children are so tied to their families, the source of the trauma is often family-related as can be seen from the cases presented above. Often the restoration of family stability after the child's perceptions of having lost that stability will begin to ameliorate the child's distress. Nevertheless, there are theorists who adhere to the position that in many cases, family intervention is a promising way of dealing with secondary trauma (e.g., Figley, 1989; Figley & Kiser, 2013; Williams, 1998).

Williams (1998, p. 119) proposes four stages for treating traumatized children: encounter and education, exploration of trauma and its impact, empowerment through skill building, and evaluation and termination. The elaboration of these stages can be found in Williams (1998), and what is presented here is a summary of what the stages involve.

In the encounter and education phase, the therapist works with the family so that all members can come to an understanding of the nature of trauma and PTSD and how their family has been impacted. Some children find this phase to be validating, while others may see themselves as victims. Either way, the therapist attempts to validate each family member's feelings and tries to get them to see how the family has been impacted. A second component here is to assure the safety of all concerned regardless of what may have taken place and to provide assurance that no negative consequences will befall anyone because of participation in therapy (e.g., Figley, 1989; Williams, 1998).

The next phase is exploration of the trauma and its impact on the family. During this second phase, "the parent reveals what he or she decides the family and others need to know about the trauma history" (Williams, 1998, p. 121). This is particularly relevant in cases of abuse where parents must exercise discretion regarding how threatening or hurtful such information might be to a given child. Therapists can assist parents in providing information that will not overwhelm the child.

Phase 3 involves empowerment and skill building. Here, among other things, the therapist helps children and other family members to develop communication skills. Children are encouraged to describe their feeling in an open and forthright manner and should receive family support for doing so. This will give the child a sense that they can be active in making change in their situation, that they have a voice in moving the family forward. The goal here is to empower children and to work against their seeing themselves as helpless victims.

The last phase is evaluation, integration, and termination. In this phase individual family members develop a perspective on where they were at the start of therapy and where they are now. The family develops a "healing theory" (Figley, 1989), which essentially involves an understanding of what happened, how it was dealt with, and how this information might be of service to others. Sometimes survivors of trauma can engage in altruistic acts such as engagement in "hotlines," or finding a new vocation to help others or presenting information on trauma recovery to classmates by way of school presentations. Children should be involved in all phases of the family healing process. "When children are kept in the dark and are not educated about trauma and the and the trauma history of a family member; when they are not included in therapy and integrated into the safe world of the trauma survivor; and when their own issues concerning power, intimacy, abuse, esteem, trust, and safety are not explored and treated, true healing for both the individual and the family system will not occur … The ultimate goal of treatment is to build resilience" (Williams, 1998, p. 128). This building of resilience applies to the family as a whole and to the individual members of the family. Children are an integral part of the family, and they and their family grow and develop resilience together as part of the therapeutic process.

## 2.14 Summary

There are many sources of childhood secondary traumatization, but one of the common elements producing this distress appears to be a perceived disruption in what the child had customarily expected life to be like. Children react to these changes as if a loss has occurred and they yearn to return to a prior status quo. Some of the many sources of this sense of loss include loss of emotional support of parental figures, witnessing parental trauma, encountering suicides, and parental reactions to war, to natural disasters, to the intergenerational transmission of trauma, to frightening imagery presented in the media, and many others. Often the restoration of the prior environment to which the child has been accustomed will result in a relatively rapid amelioration of the child's distress. Nevertheless, children, very much like adults, acquire the distress of parental or other caregiving figures and as a result suffer secondary trauma reactions. Treatments can involve family therapy as the child's trauma most often develops within the family context. For that reason, family intervention is frequently called for, and the goal of this intervention is to empower family members and to strengthen their resilience.

# Chapter 3
# Adult Family Caregivers

The major source of secondary traumatization occurs within families especially when parents and siblings must support an ailing or otherwise traumatized family member. In fact, it is estimated that family caregivers represent approximately 20% of the US adult population (American Association of Retired Persons [AARP] and National Alliance for Caregiving [NAC], 2020). The stresses and emotional demands of such caregiving can be considerable regardless of whether the family member's illness is due to physical, emotional, or cognitive dysfunction or some combination of these (Shulz et al., 2020). It is not uncommon for caregivers to experience elevated levels of depression, anxiety, emotional and physical exhaustion, increases in financial worries, and an exacerbation of their own underlying illnesses due to the stresses and emotional demands placed on them. Given the significance of secondary trauma within families, this chapter will present three such cases in depth.

One of the sources of secondary traumatic stress within families involves the caring for those who have been sickened by the COVID-19 virus (Dorn et al., 2020). Beach et al. (2021) conducted a cross-sectional study comparing caregivers to non-caregivers during the COVID pandemic. Family caregivers reported increased duties and burdens resulting in adverse health, psychological, and financial problems. Compared to non-caregivers, caregivers had elevated anxiety, depression, fatigue, sleep disturbance, and loneliness. Similarly, 27% of parents of school-age children who had been diagnosed with COVID-19 reported worsening mental health for themselves, and 14% reported a deterioration of the mental health of their children (Garbe et al., 2020). At the time of this writing, the novel coronavirus, which appears to have begun in the USA in 2019 (COVID-19), has been responsible for over 900 thousand deaths in the USA alone and more than 6 million deaths worldwide. In addition to these deaths, there are untold numbers of people who now test negative for COVID-19 following infection and yet continue to have a variety of physical and psychological symptoms such as fatigue, breathing problems, impaired sense of taste and smell, and psychological difficulties such as anxiety and

© The Author(s), under exclusive license to Springer Nature Switzerland AG 2023

R. W. Motta, *Secondary Trauma*, https://doi.org/10.1007/978-3-031-44308-4_3

depression. They are called “long haulers” because they continue to have COVID-related symptoms long after the virus is no longer detectable in their systems.

## 3.1 Case 1: Jordan and the Family Pain of Living with a Long Hauler

Jordan and his family were, and continue to be, significantly impacted by what is believed to be a COVID-19 infection. Jordan’s symptoms include experiencing shortness of breath, fatigue, and overwhelming, long-running panic attacks, which to him are the most distressing of his symptoms. His panic attacks frequently result in extreme agitation, thrashing about, destroying objects, and even attacking people. His mother and sister have endured secondary traumatization that evolves from taking care of a sick family member and sharing his pain and distress. They are especially troubled by the extreme irrationality and occasional physical aggressiveness that occur in conjunction with the panic attacks.

Jordan is an adjunct psychology professor who has also provided psychological services to school systems. He is 51, single, and often lives with his mother and sister although he also has his own apartment. Prior to his viral infection, Jordan had sought counseling for comparatively mild depression and self-doubt related to vocational difficulties. Aside from these relatively minor difficulties, he was socially engaged, content, and had an active dating life. His fraternal twin sister is a successful computer consultant who is a co-owner of a profitable company that provides Internet and cloud security services to international banks.

Jordan’s mother, who is now 75, was infected with the COVID-19 virus at age 73. She experienced extreme pain, exhaustion, and breathing difficulties, and these problems went on for more than a year. While symptoms of COVID-19 typically resolve in a few weeks or months, her difficulties continued, perhaps since she also had underlying lupus erythematosus, an autoimmune disorder, prior to being infected with the virus. According to attending physicians, Jordan’s mother appears to have infected her son with the virus although his symptoms were initially said to be so mild as to be undetected and not warranting intervention. These physicians maintain that despite his mild symptoms and initially negative COVID test results, Jordan appears to have developed some form of neurologically based difficulty that manifests itself in extreme agitation and prolonged panic attacks, and these appear to be related to COVID infection. The physicians, after more than a year of attempting to understand Jordan’s symptoms, gave him a spinal tap, the results of which provided some clarification of Jordan’s condition. The neurologists involved with his case concluded that the panic reactions were the result of a condition referred to autoimmune encephalitis, whereby healthy brain tissue is attacked by one’s own immune system. While the specific origin of the panic attacks remains unclear, his doctors have speculated that Jordan’s immune system misinterprets the presence of a pathogen existing in the nervous system and attacks that system. The nervous system is then said to react with panic as a behavioral manifestation of being attacked. Over time a neural cycle begins to build such that panic attacks are immediately set off at any hint of the central nervous system being impacted by the immune system (Butler & Moseley, 2015).

Jordan's agitation and panic have, as of this writing, persisted for almost 2 years. He feels tormented by overwhelming anxiety, which he claims can last for hours and is worse in the mornings. Typical panic attacks last about 10–15 min. He has reported that there are times when his panic will last for most of the day. He is taking antidepressants and antianxiety medications along with anti-inflammatory drugs and immunoglobulin under the presumption that his brain has become inflamed because of autoimmune encephalitis and the over-reactivity of the immune system. At one point Jordan's agitation and anxiety became so extreme that he attempted suicide by throwing himself into traffic from a moving car and by attempting to throw himself off the porch of his sister's apartment. He has been hospitalized in five different psychiatric facilities due to his irrational behavior. Each time, his symptoms seemed to get worse as a result of being in a hospital environment. Attending physicians would then release him on the presumption that the hospital environment exacerbated his difficulties. On more than one occasion, he would simply escape from the psychiatric facility and flee into the streets. At no point has he been diagnosed as psychotic although some of his verbalizations involving a delusion of brain entrapment inside of his skull seem psychotic-like. He is presently being seen by a psychologist, psychiatrist, physical therapist, a nutritionist, and his health aide and has received long hauler outpatient services at Mount Sinai Hospital and Lennox Hill Hospital in New York City where the focus of intervention has been on dealing with presumed dysautonomia, a dysfunction of the autonomic nervous system. The rehabilitation specialists at Mount Sinai saw his panic attacks as behavioral manifestations of brain inflammation (Butler & Moseley, 2015). As of this writing, Jordan has been in several hospitals and psychiatric facilities from which he has fled or been discharged and is now on a locked ward at Lennox Hill Hospital in Manhattan. His symptoms appear to be little improved despite the positive expectations of his physicians.

In counseling sessions Jordan relates that he becomes overwhelmed by panic attacks, particularly in the morning. He reports an extremely painful phobic reaction involving the fear that "my brain is trapped in my skull." While this statement seems to have an irrational or even psychotic ring to it, Jordan does not show the disorders of thought that are typically associated with psychotic processes.

It is difficult to convey the level of psychological pain that Jordan experiences during one of his routine panic attacks. He describes the attacks as "seizures," during which he is overcome by indescribably intense and irrational fear. While enduring one of these attacks, he will thrash around in what looks like maniacal spasms. Sometimes he will physically assault family members and his health aide, while also destroying objects within his reach. In one of these episodes, he punched his mother in the face and seemed unaware of it the next day. In fact, he asked her if she had fallen as her eye was swollen. During therapy sessions he will cry out in agony, stating, "I can't take this anymore. My life is ruined," and will also make suicidal threats. In the time that he has been suffering, he has shown some minimal level of improvement, but overall, he remains dramatically impaired, suffering, and unable to work. There is little question that Jordan is enduring intensely traumatic experiences, and as a result his mother and sister are secondarily traumatized to a significant degree. Jordan's impairment has caused considerable secondary traumatic stress for his family.

Jordan's mother agonizes over the fact that she may have inadvertently caused Jordan's pain by possibly infecting him with the virus she was carrying. She carries extreme guilt over her view that she may have been responsible for "ruining my son's life." Her world has become disrupted, and she seems to be unable to obtain any pleasure in living. She is tormented by her son's intense suffering and lives in constant fear that he will hurt himself or put an end to his life. She has verbalized that she feels so tortured by her son's disability that it is likely to cause her death. Recently Jordan jumped from a set of stairs while staying with his mother and sister and broke bones in his foot. This behavior can be viewed a quasi-suicidal or "parasuicidal" gesture. It is an expression of Jordan's extreme torment and his ambivalence about killing himself. After all, if he really intended to kill himself, he would have done so. Either way, his mother suffers in seeing her son suffering, and this is typical of secondary traumatization. She describes her feelings as "pain beyond imagining."

Jordan's sister is also experiencing secondary trauma in that most of her waking moments are taken up with trying to find health-care professionals or programs to help her brother, while living with the gnawing fear that all will fail and Jordan will kill himself. "This is my twin brother. I have to do all I am humanly capable of to save him." Her life is absorbed with assuring her brother's well-being, and she experiences intense anxiety that all her efforts will fail. There is room for little else in her life except, of course, her concerns about her mother. She worries that the stress that is being placed on her mother will be life-threatening given that her mother is 75 and is weakened by lupus. Jordan's sister has been so overburdened, so secondarily traumatized, that she too shows panic attacks and lapses into frantic cries stating that no one can help her and that she is all alone in her efforts to find help for her brother. Her frantic efforts to "guide" Jordan's doctors have resulted in their wanting to distance themselves from her. They view her well-meaning efforts as interfering with Jordan's treatment and as calling into question their ability to provide care for him.

While this case may appear extreme, it is typical of situations in which secondary traumatization occurs because of the illness of a family member. The ailing person suffers, and the family is "infected" in such a way that the suffering becomes communal. Jordan experiences severe bouts of panic and endures major depression over thoughts such as "my life is over" and "I will never return to my previous life." Comments like these are torturous for loving family members who do all they can to reduce their loved one's pain. The family lives with the dreadful fear that the afflicted family member may not get better and may commit suicide, and as a result they experience extreme distress. They suffer along with the sufferer. While it is true that Jordan's life has been disrupted, it is equally true that his sister's and mother's lives have also been radically upended. His sister is unable to work and lives with constant anxiety and unhappiness over what she sees in her brother while also being preoccupied with her mother's well-being. The mother experiences a combination of guilt, profound sadness, and fear that her son may not get better and may even kill himself and that it might be her fault. Theirs is a hellish existence by anyone's definition. All family members dread what the next day may bring. They lead a tormented daily ritual.

Family members suffer regardless of whether the ailing member is enduring a physical illness, a severe dysfunction such as schizophrenia or bipolar disorder, an unrelenting eating disorder, or various forms of traumatic experiences. The case of Jordan highlights secondary trauma due to a suspected COVID infection, which may or may not have been the stimulus for the presence of autoimmune encephalitis, but again, it is not unique. This case is ongoing and there is no resolution. However, the rehabilitation services that Jordan is receiving seem to be causing the panic attacks to become ever so slightly less severe and less prolonged. These improvements may bode well for the future for both Jordan and his mother and sister, but for the present their pain continues unabated. Their despair, exhaustion, and preoccupation with Jordan are characteristics of secondary traumatization within families.

The following case, unlike the case of Jordan, is of an assaulted and traumatized family member whose individual trauma became a family trauma.

## 3.2 Case 2: The Swimmer's Family Suffers Her Rape

Ellen's primary traumatic experiences were previously addressed in detail (Motta, 2021), and here the major focus will be on the secondary traumatization encountered by her family. Ellen's mother and father describe her as having been "the perfect child." She was attractive, an excellent student, courteous, loving, outgoing, and highly disciplined. Regardless of whether Ellen was preparing for exams or for a swim meet, she was focused and always prepared assiduously. She became a cheerleader in high school, while also being an outstanding and award-winning swimmer. She was the editor of the school newspaper and maintained a straight-A average. Her father had served in the Vietnam War and had spent 10 years in the army as a noncommissioned officer. His wish was for his daughter to attend one of the military academies, preferably West Point because that was the service academy dedicated to producing the army's future officers. Ellen wished to please her father and did apply, and was accepted, to West Point, but she also was accepted to a university in California which, although lacking in the acclaim of a military academy, had a top-tier swimming program that had produced more than one Olympic hopeful. Ellen chose to pursue her Olympic dreams in California, and although the school was not her father's first choice, he was nevertheless proud that his daughter would pursue her dream with her usual ferocious determination.

As was typical of her, Ellen threw herself into her studies and was maintaining the A average to which she and her family had been accustomed. But it was swimming and swimming-related exercise that consumed most of Ellen's time and effort. Six hours of each day, 6 days a week, were dedicated to swimming laps and strength training. She would rise early in the morning and troop off to the pool where she would put in 1–3 h before the start of classes. After classes it was back to the pool or off to the gym for resistance and flexibility training. As she did in high school, Ellen once again attracted the attention of her coaches with her numerous wins at intercollegiate swim meets. Her coaches saw her Olympic potential and Ellen pursued this goal with single-minded tenacity. Back home her parents were filled with pride over the continued accomplishments of their daughter.

All seemed to be going just as Ellen had planned until an end-of-year fraternity party put an end to her dreams. She attended this party with two of her girlfriends from her swim team. The two friends and Ellen were drinking beer, but not excessively, and were enjoying the stress-relieving party atmosphere. Two muscled male water polo team players from her school invited Ellen into a room to show her some of the awards their team had won. When Ellen went into the room, the door was shut behind her, and two events occurred, both of which destroyed all she had worked for.

These athletic young men grabbed her and pinned her arms and legs while forcibly removing her clothing. With one holding her down, the other raped her, and then they switched roles so that each had a turn with her. Ellen's mind could not comprehend what was happening. She was so overwhelmed that she entered a dissociative state where she almost felt as if she were viewing a young woman being raped rather than being raped herself. This was without a doubt a horrible situation, but the second event that tormented Ellen even more than the rape was the fact that she did not fight off her attackers. Despite her strength and fitness, she made no effort to aggressively defend herself. She did not scream for help, nor did she resist in any way. She simply went limp while her attackers assaulted her. This "freeze" response is often seen in the animal world when one animal is overwhelmed by a stronger predator (Levine, 2010). The attacked animal goes into a frozen, seemingly dead state. It is theorized that this might be a last defense as many predators do not seek out the dead as a food source. The fight, flight, and freeze responses are known characteristics of the sympathetic nervous system. Ellen froze in response to her assault, and it was this freeze response, this passivity in the face of an attack, that caused both extreme distress and confusion. She simply could not understand why she did not defend herself.

Ellen made it back to her dorm in a dazed and frenzied state. She did not attend classes the next day. She isolated herself and, for the first time in her life, began to drink heavily and started using cocaine. While still enrolled at school, she no longer attended classes, nor did she participate in her swimming activities. Shortly after the official ending of the semester, she made her way to her parents' home and withdrew into her room. Her parents were stunned to see the radical change in their daughter. Despite repeated efforts they were unable to get Ellen to communicate with them. She was hostile, avoidant, and altogether a radically altered person.

These self-alterations are common in virtually all forms of trauma and PTSD (Motta, 2021). Ellen was drinking heavily, was using illicit drugs, and began smoking cigarettes. Her parents found cocaine in her room and at that point insisted that she enter therapy or leave home.

At first Ellen's parents tried to be supportive as they could clearly see that something had happened to their daughter and that she was in distress. Their efforts to be supportive were repeatedly rebuffed as were their efforts to try to find out what had happened at school. They felt powerless and preoccupied with their daughter's radically uncharacteristic behavior. It was out of severe disappointment over the loss of the daughter they once knew and frustration over her violations of the rules of the house including her drinking, smoking, and drug use that they gave her an ultimatum to get help or leave home. Like many of the cases involving secondary traumatization that have been covered to this point, there was a sense of loss. In this case it was a loss of the daughter they had known and loved for many years. Her pain became their pain. Her irritability and sadness became theirs. The major difference between Ellen and her parents was that Ellen knew why she was reacting the way she did, but her withdrawal left her parents confused, overwhelmed, and not knowing which way to turn.

Ellen's parents experienced a gnawing emptiness, which appeared like a grief reaction that might be seen in the death of a family member. In many ways there had been a loss. Ellen, although physically present, was not the same Ellen that they knew and loved. The transformed Ellen was diametrically opposite to the one they knew. The prior Ellen was loving, open, accomplished, and focused. This one was remote, withdrawn, angry, drug-taking, and lacking in any sense of direction. A crime had been committed involving Ellen, but that crime also impacted her family. Ellen was keenly aware that her problem behavior was negatively impacting her family and was troubled that their upset may have absorbed them to such an extent that her own troubles were becoming less important. For this reason, "survivors often hesitate to disclose to family members, not only because they fear they will not be understood but also because they fear that the reactions of the family members will overshadow their own" (Herman, 1992, p. 65).

At the start of therapy, Ellen was resistant to revealing what had taken place and would simply blame her parents' "nosiness and demands on me" as the reason for her negativity. Ultimately, she did reveal what took place, and it was clear that her drugging and drinking were her way of anesthetizing the pain of her rape and her inability to comprehend why she had not put up a fight when being assaulted. After several attempts the therapist was able to convince Ellen to bring her parents into the session and to share what had taken place. This involvement of her family had a significantly positive impact on all concerned. Ellen was relieved of the great weight of bearing her pain alone, and her parents finally were able to make sense of what was taking place.

As in other cases of secondary trauma, Ellen's pain was also shouldered by her parents, and they not only wanted to help their daughter overcome her difficulties and move on with her life, but they also sought retribution and restitution. Specifically, they wanted Ellen to testify in court, have her attackers jailed, and have her school refund tuition. Their reasoning for seeking the refund was that they had paid tens of thousands of dollars to send their child to a school that placed their daughter in an assaultive environment. More than the return of tuition, they wanted retribution. Ellen's rapists had taken the daughter they knew from them, and they wanted the attackers to pay dearly. The attackers hurt them as parents, and they wanted payback. Unfortunately, much as her parents wanted punishment for the rapists, Ellen adamantly refused to go to the police and file the necessary complaint. This was terribly frustrating for the parents who felt that in a way they too had been raped. The attackers had violated their daughter and their sense of family. Despite all of this, Ellen felt that going to the police and then to court would force her to relive her torment, and she feared that nothing would come of it. Unfortunately, she may have been right.

The statistics regarding the outcome of rape reporting are not encouraging. Herman (1992) claims that approximately one-third of women report having been sexually assaulted at some time in their lives and one-quarter report having been raped. Of the latter group, approximately one in ten will report the incident to the police. After a police report, only 1 in 100 cases will result in an arrest and 1 in 200 in a conviction of some kind. One might think that in today's world these grim statistics may have improved since the time Herman reported them and that those who are raped now have a better chance of receiving justice. Carnigella (2009), however, suggests that the statistics reported above may be a conservative estimate of what is taking place. Carnigella indicates that in most rapes, far fewer than the one in ten presented by Herman (1992) will ever be reported to police and because of this, the crime of rape is one of those societal transgressions for which the possibility of being punished is remarkably low. While the US courts may provide more justice than is seen in many patriarchal and third-world countries, rape continues to be a crime for which the probability of punishment is often vanishingly small.

## 3.3 Ellen's Parents Are Impacted by Secondary Trauma

Ellen's demoralized parents were finally able to get some level of retribution in that the school terminated the enrollment of the two accused rapists. In addition, they were able to get the last semester's tuition returned to them. But without Ellen's going to the police to report a rape, nothing more could be accomplished. By their own account, Ellen's parents felt that they too had been raped. A terrible injustice had occurred to their beloved daughter, and this caused her to be transformed into a being that they no longer knew. Their sense of loss was profound. They felt as if someone had entered this tight-knit family and ripped it apart. They felt intense anxiety as a result of not knowing what was to become of their daughter, depression over the unfairness of the situation and seeing a loved one severely hurt and impaired, feelings of isolation because they were reluctant to share what had happened to any of their friends or other more distant family members, and powerless and helplessness because there was little they could do make the situation better. Their thoughts were constantly intruded upon by memories of the miserable situation in which the family now found itself. They were distracted and had difficulty concentrating because of their preoccupation with their daughter. They also felt a deep sense of shame, which in many ways mirrored the debasement that Ellen felt in having been treated as an object upon whom sexual and aggressive urges had been meted out. Ellen had been assaulted and felt powerless. Owing to secondary traumatization, Ellen's parents felt the same way—assaulted and powerless.

## 3.4 Recovery

The process of recovery was slow, but it did occur. As a result of family therapy, both Ellen and her parents were able to express their feelings and to slowly begin to restore the love and support that had been hallmarks of their family. While Ellen continued to refuse to go to the police and to the courts to seek justice, she reengaged her focus and determination and decided to transfer her college credits to a local institution and major in psychology. She now went at her academics with the same ferocity and focus that she had displayed in the past, but where previously her goals had involved swimming, they now involved helping other female students who had been assaulted. Throughout her college years, she was involved in sexual assault organizations and began giving talks at local high schools. She became a sought-out speaker because of the power of her firsthand experience and the articulate and sensitive way she was able to present herself.

Just as illness and trauma negatively impact the entire family, the recovery from trauma can also help the family heal. Ellen's single-minded determination to turn her traumatic experience into a resource that could be used to help others became a catalyst that helped her parents to also begin seeing things in a more positive light. They encouraged their daughter to continue her high school sexual assault talks and began making their own contacts with surrounding schools to get them to invite Ellen to do presentations. The road to recovery was slow for this family, but they were able to take a terrible event and transform it into something that could benefit society. Ellen continued in therapy and over time was able to become a more thoughtful and balanced individual. Her parents became more engaged in their community and with programs designed to help victims of sexual assault. They were also able to begin to enjoy family travel and vacations, all of which helped them heal. While this case resulted in a positive outcome, there are many who are severely, and to some extent permanently, damaged by situations such as Ellen's. The nineteenth-century philosopher Friedrich Nietzsche might have stated that what does not kill me makes me stronger, but in many instances, people experience long-running damage owing to their traumatic experiences, and their families are also damaged through the process of secondary traumatization.

## 3.5 Case 3: Rob and Laura Receive Shocking News

Rob had graduated from college in the early 1990s and then volunteered to serve in the US Army for reasons that he is not sure of, but he states that it might have been a combination of excitement seeking and patriotism. After basic and advanced infantry training, he was sent to Iraq and participated in a developing war. The Iraqi war appears to have been started when the Iraqi leader Saddam Hussein took the provocative and questionable stance that neighboring Kuwait was siphoning off Iraqi oil. This resulted in Iraq's invasion of Kuwait and the subsequent involvement of US combat forces. After having engaged in a few nightmarish combat assaults, Rob decided that he had to make something of his life if he ever got through the war alive. While still in Iraq, he applied and was accepted to a graduate degree program back in the US that trained school guidance counselors. While attending classes and while also receiving psychotherapy for war-related PTSD, Rob met Laura, who worked as the secretary to the counseling department chair. Laura was married to an alcoholic and abusive husband. A chemistry developed between Rob and Laura possibly because they may have seen each other as a positive and dramatic contrast to the troubled lives they were currently living. After a few dates, Rob and Laura were becoming deeply attached to each other, and it was during this time that Laura finally decided to leave her abusive husband. They continued dating even after Rob finished his graduate program and became employed as a guidance counselor in a local school district.

Rob bought his first house and Laura subsequently agreed to move in with him. They lived together for 4 years, and one day Rob worked up the courage to ask Laura to marry him. Although she was content with their living arrangements, she believed that marrying Rob was the right thing to do if she were to fulfill her unstated dream of having a baby. Rob and Laura married, and after a year of trying, there was no pregnancy, and they both agreed to go to a fertility specialist to see if either of them had any medical issues that might interfere with a pregnancy. After a thorough medical evaluation, Laura was told that she had a "tipped" uterus, and this may have contributed to the pregnancy difficulties. A tiny cyst was also found on her left breast and the fertility specialist suggested that she have it biopsied. He assured Laura that he was almost certain that the cyst was nothing to be concerned about and that these breast cysts were commonly seen.

Rob took Laura for the biopsy, and he paced expectantly in the waiting room while the procedure was being performed. The surgeon who conducted the biopsy looked glum as he came out of surgery to meet with Rob. The news could not have been worse. The surgeon stated that although he needed confirmation from pathology, what looked like a cyst to the fertility specialist had all the earmarks of cancer. At this point Rob remembers having a sense of what is called "derealization" in the psychological literature. It is an otherworldly experience that sometimes follows traumatic and shocking events. This news simply did not fit into the world as Rob knew it or expected it to be. It is as if he were receiving information from an alien world. The resulting pathology report did show that the "cyst" was breast cancer, and so began Rob and Laura's confrontation with both primary and secondary traumas.

Rob vowed to Laura that he would do everything within his power to support her as they sought out treatment. And as it turned out, there were many such treatments. Doctors at New York University Medical Center, Sloane Kettering Cancer Center, and Stoneybrook State University of New York Medical Center tried everything from surgery, to radiation, to experimental high-dose chemotherapy, and to immunotherapy. At times it appeared that the cancer was in remission, and then it would dishearteningly reappear, and it began to spread to other areas of her body.

Laura's treatments involved several hospitalizations, tormenting nausea due to chemotherapy, and days on the couch in utter exhaustion and general malaise. Their lives had been transformed from hopeful expectation of starting a family to ongoing dread and fear. Rob and Laura confronted this adversity with courage and a refusal to give up hope. Nevertheless, the burdens they were carrying were wearying to both. When able, Laura would occupy herself with gardening, although her oncologist advised against this as her immune system was weakened by chemotherapy and there were concerns about infections. Laura also tried to keep her many friendships alive and well although she often lacked the energy to do so. Rob stayed busy with work and with running to hospitals, coordinating treatments, and speaking with physicians. Although trying to stay focused, he was tormented by watching the suffering of his beloved wife. This couple tried to maintain their humor in the face of adversity and often joked with each other that Laura resembled a "martian" after the chemotherapy caused all her hair to fall out.

Laura fought her disease courageously and tried not to acknowledge the fear of impending death. Rob, although always enjoying his time with Laura, suffered an aloneness and a gnawing ever-present sense of dread. His secondary traumatization along with his PTSD from his war experiences was taking their toll. "Imagine a rat inside your stomach, gnawing your insides. That is how I feel most of the time," he glumly stated. His only relief was sleep where the dread he was living with would temporarily abate. And then he would awaken and realize that he was back in a hellish world of struggle to survive and an enduring fear that the end was inevitable. While Laura kept up with her friends and gardening activities, Rob continued to immerse himself in work, exercise, and meditation in addition to coordinating Laura's treatments. His meditations focused on tranquility and expectancy of a positive outcome for Laura. All these activities served as distractors and ways of coping with his gnawing fears. Laura was dealing with the primary trauma of living with what appeared to be a lethal disease. Rob was secondarily traumatized by what was happening to Laura physically and emotionally. Her distress was his too.

After a Christmas celebration with Rob and her family, Laura was having difficulty breathing, was constantly coughing, felt utterly exhausted, and was taken to the hospital. This was the 10th year of Rob and Laura's marriage, and for 9 of these years, they had struggled with cancer. The initial diagnosis following Laura's hospitalization was that she had pneumonia. But, after a series of scans and blood tests, it was determined that in addition to pneumonia, she also had lung cancer. Further testing ensued and the findings were that the cancer had not only spread to her lungs but also to her brain, liver, and multiple areas of her bones, especially in her legs, pelvis, and spine. To quote the attending oncologist's grimly delivered diagnosis, "Her situation is hopeless." "Hopeless" was not a word that Rob and Laura ever allowed themselves to consider. Shortly after this bleak prognosis, Laura began to slip into a state of diminishing consciousness. All cancer treatment had been stopped, and the only medication she was receiving was morphine to cope with the pain that the cancer of the bones brought on.

In addition to the ongoing secondary traumatization that Rob had been enduring for years, he reported a searingly painful memory that he says will always be with him. At one point, while Laura appeared to be in a coma, a physician informed Rob that Laura was simply in a lower level of consciousness but was not in a coma. He demonstrated this by loudly calling Laura's name and demanding that she wake up. Her eyes did open and at that point the physician pointed to Rob and loudly asked Laura, "Do you know this man?" She looked directly at Rob and shook her head indicating that she did not know him. While this exercise proved the physician's point about consciousness, it was "A knife in my heart," said Rob. It was clear that the woman whom he loved so deeply, although still alive, was lost forever. The cancer in her brain had caused irreparable damage. One week after this dispiriting and traumatic experience, Laura died with Rob and her parents at her bedside.

## 3.6 Grief and Recovery

Rob's secondary trauma, his shared and silent suffering over the distress that Laura was enduring, had ended. He now moved into the searing pain of grief and felt as if he were dead inside. The once colorful world he shared with Laura was now gray and lifeless. He was living in an emotional desert despite having sought out grief counseling. With time, Rob made slow and uneven progress in pulling his life back together. He began dating a year after Laura's death, but none of his efforts led to anything meaningful. One day Rob was speaking to Anna, a guidance counselor in a neighboring school district about a troubled boy who was transferring from Rob's district to hers. Rob was impressed with Anna's sensitivity and deeply felt compassion for the students she worked with and after several phone conversations; he asked her out to dinner. The dinner turned out to be unexpectedly magical. There was an instant and obvious mutual connection between them. They shared many of the same interests including a love of nature and the outdoors, and they began dating regularly. They became exclusive and inseparable lovers for 5 years. It became obvious that they could not be away from each other, and eventually Rob asked Anna to marry him right after they had completed a long and arduous trek to the top of Pike's Peak in Colorado. Anna said yes to Rob's proposal and they both sobbed with joy. Rob later joked that Anna was confused by the cold temperature and lower level of oxygen at the top of this big mountain, and that is why she agreed to marry him.

Rob and Anna are now living a joyful life together and although they do not have their own child, Rob happily inherited a wonderful stepson and stepdaughter from Anna's previous marriage. Rob's searingly painful past has finally been put to rest, and he has moved on to a new life and new beginnings with a compassionate and loving companion. What this case clearly shows is that secondary trauma is a seemingly necessary consequence of caring. One cannot be emotionally involved with others, whether it be as a family member, lover, dear friend, or as a committed health-care provider, without vicariously experiencing the other's joys and sorrows. The research in secondary trauma shows that we are tied to others, and when they suffer, we suffer and that this is especially true when the one in emotional pain is a family member (Figley, 1995), as it was here. This case and the other presented cases also show that recovery from secondary traumatic experiences does occur; that one is able to move on and make a healthy and positive adaptation following both trauma and loss.

## 3.7 Summary

The early studies of secondary or vicarious traumatization were produced by those who were professionally involved in client care (e.g., McCann & Pearlman, 1990; Pearlman & Saakvitne, 1995). This literature was relevant to psychologists, psychiatrists, social workers, and other mental health professionals, and it carefully described how the distress of clients could transfer to those who were treating them. This early emphasis on health-care providers was an important contribution to research but gave the erroneous impression that secondary trauma was primarily a form of distress or "emotional exhaustion" specifically relevant to health-care professions. We can see from this chapter and from those that follow that while secondary trauma is a common affliction of the mental health industry, it is an even greater and more pervasive problem for families. The fact that approximately one-fifth of family members are involved in caring for an ailing or otherwise traumatized relative suggests that multiple millions may experience some level of secondary trauma. The strong emotional bonds within families can result in equally strong emotional burdens when family members are in distress. The emotional ties among parents, children, siblings, and others in the family unit are far stronger than other ties, such as those to coworkers and clients, and therefore families become the major source of secondary trauma in terms of numbers and perhaps in terms of intensity. Nevertheless, there is little doubt that therapists, nurses, doctors, and others outside of the family can also be traumatized by the demands of their profession and that is the area to which we now turn.

# Chapter 4
# Secondary Trauma in Professional Caregivers

It was noted in the prior chapter that the most common source of secondary traumatization is that which occurs when family members are emotionally impacted by the suffering of another family member, regardless of whether the original sufferer was enduring a physical, emotional, or other psychiatric difficulty. Although less common than family-based secondary trauma, secondary traumatization commonly occurs among clinicians who treat the traumatized. This form of secondary trauma is so impactful that Figley (1989) expressed dismay that many clinicians who work with traumatized individuals often leave the field because they acquire their clients' emotional pain and can no longer endure the suffering of those with whom they are working. "The same kind of psychosocial mechanisms within families that make trauma 'contagious,' that create a context for family members to infect one another with their traumatic material, operate between traumatized clients and the therapist" (p. 144). Figley further maintains that those clinicians who are most vulnerable to developing secondary trauma are those who have a pronounced inclination to see themselves as saviors and rescuers. Perhaps these self-views place extra stress on clinicians when they observe that those for whom they care are not significantly improving or are moving too slowly. The lack of progress may serve to invalidate, negate, or challenge their self-view as a rescuer.

McCann and Pearlman (1990) produced seminal reports on the secondary traumatic impact on psychotherapists who treat the traumatized and their findings are also relevant to those providers whose involvements might be primarily of a medical or rehabilitative nature. They coined the term *vicarious traumatization* to describe the secondary trauma seen in health-care providers who work with traumatized individuals. These care providers reportedly begin to incorporate into their own view of life those schemata maintained by the clients they are treating. For example, those who work primarily with rape victims who are understandably wary of their environments may begin to incorporate the fear, suspicion, and depressive effects of the victims they treat. These health-care providers may develop nightmares of rapes and have rape preoccupations intrude upon them unexpectedly. They can also develop a

© The Author(s), under exclusive license to Springer Nature Switzerland AG 2023

R. W. Motta, *Secondary Trauma*, https://doi.org/10.1007/978-3-031-44308-4_4

general wariness and distrust of the environment and a hesitant and self-protective emotional reluctance to initiate and act reciprocally in relationships. Social isolation and an increasing use of alcohol and drugs may be attempts to lower exposure to trauma material, and the alcohol and drugs might also be used in excess to dampen painful memories.

## 4.1 Secondary Trauma and Medical Care

A typical example of the negative impact that can befall health-care providers can be seen in the report of a young internist who was completing her residency at a hospital with a heavy caseload of severely ill COVID patients. She remarked, "People say I'm a hero for doing this work. I'm not. I'm disrupted and tormented by the suffering of my patients. I'm also in constant fear that I will be infected and bring the virus home to my one-year-old son. If it were up to me, I would flee this hospital" (J. Manley, personal communication, June 19, 2020).

A detailed personal account of the unique stress experienced by nurses is presented by Wright (2016). This deeply compassionate health-care provider's journey into the dark world of secondary trauma began with the statement, "He was flatline when they brought him in.... Seventeen-year-old male in an MVA" (p. 1). That event took place 10 years earlier, but she states that in her mind it could have taken place today. It is among the many memories that ate at her. There was nothing she could do for this car accident victim, nor could she ameliorate her feeling of helplessness in dealing with the situation. She continued to encounter emotionally debilitating experiences on a regular basis because of constant exposure to, and inability to relieve, the suffering of her patients. Regarding STS (secondary traumatic stress), she states, "With repeated exposure to the suffering of others, symptoms progress until the condition is almost indistinguishable from PTSD." She further reports that "A loss of joy, withdrawal from intimacy, episodes of depression, and even suicide, are all possible" (p. 37) because of secondary traumatic experiences. Her personal observations sum up nicely the consequences of the emotional drain and the demands on health-care professionals inherent in the caring for others. In order to cope with her STS, she engaged in a series of ultimately unsuccessful activities including psychotherapy, eye movement desensitization and reprocessing (EMDR; Shapiro, 2001), yoga, psychotropic medication, meditation, reiki, chiropractic, cruises, immersion in nature, shamanism, writing courses, and other interventions. All these interventions helped to some degree but not to the extent that they significantly reduced her emotional pain and joyless existence. Ultimately the only activity that helped her to any substantial and lasting degree was leaving her career. She considered herself lucky in that she did not commit suicide.

Wright's autographical account and Figley's (1989) dismay over providers leaving the field provide clear insights into how draining and exhausting secondary trauma from health service provision can be. The stressors eventually wear away at an individual. The term *compassion fatigue* (Figley, 1995) is a simple expression that captures the secondary traumatic process well. The stress of helping others eventually wears one down. They are fatigued and drained both emotionally and physically. Often the only avenue that provides relief is leaving the field or in some extreme instances, taking of one's life.

Dr. Lorna Breen's case was chronicled by *The New York Times* (Watkins et al., 2020). Dr. Breen was the medical director of the emergency department of New York-Presbyterian Allen Hospital in Manhattan, New York, where she had a heavy caseload of severely ill COVID patients. Despite her burdensome job demands she had been described by colleagues as upbeat and energetic. She was said to always be looking out for the needs of others, especially in making sure that her medical personnel had protective equipment and whatever else they needed in the hospital to do their jobs effectively. Her family reported that she had no history of mental illness and in fact was extroverted, socially engaged, and regularly traveled out west to snowboard and ski. At the time, April 2020, New York was the epicenter in the US of severe COVID cases, and as of April 7, there had been 59 patient deaths at Dr. Breen's hospital. The stresses on the medical staff were intense, and it was at that time that Dr. Breen herself contracted the virus. It then appears that, although she seemed to be recovering well, the combination of the emotional stressors of working with COVID patients and her own exhaustion and decreased ability to cope with these stressors led her to take her own life. Her work was a likely contributor to "compassion fatigue," and the exhaustion and lessened ability to cope brought on by the coronavirus simply became too much for her. Nurse Wright, above, acknowledged the potential for suicide resulting from the emotional drain of nursing. These demands and the COVID virus simply overwhelmed Dr. Breen, a physician who otherwise seemed remarkably capable of withstanding the stressors of her work.

In another such case, Chaz related the personal emotional difficulties he encountered while working as a physician's assistant in the Bronx, New York, for 19 years (personal communication, August 10, 2021). Chaz stated that the clinic in which he worked was often inundated with emergencies resulting from car accidents, assaults, and muggings, in addition to the usual sprains, colds, and flu. The intensity of his work often left him depressed and feeling emotionally depleted. He dealt with these stressors by exercising and found bicycling to be a particularly healthy way to reduce his distress. Fly fishing was also a way of escaping the ongoing job pressures, and he stated that these escapes allowed him to continue with his job.

One Tuesday morning in September 2001, Chaz was driving to work when his car was avalanched by thunderous falling debris from the New York City World Trade Center terrorist attack. The vehicle was crushed, and he sustained serious foot and hip injuries, which required months of physical therapy. Oddly, it was not this shocking situation that pushed him to leave his employment. Rather, it was a subsequent event that he encountered that was the proverbial final straw for him. After his recovery from the foot and hip injuries, he was called upon to respond to an emergency in a subway station where it was reported that someone had either jumped or was pushed onto the tracks of an oncoming train. He expected that he would find a seriously injured person, or worse, but on arrival he looked down at the tracks and saw only a bloody shoe. There was nothing else. The victim had been crushed by the train and pulled along underneath it. The parents of the victim were soon called and came to the station. They wanted to meet with Chaz to see what he knew, but he was unable to provide any concrete information. Their intense and inconsolable despair left Chaz deeply shaken. He could not stop ruminating over how he would feel if this tragedy had happened to his own daughter. His usual diversions for managing his emotional distress seemed to be of no use to him. Figley (1989) had lamented the fact that many health-care workers leave their fields because of the emotional demands of their work, and this is what happened with Chaz. It was not his own injuries from the terrorist attack on the World Trade Center that finally pushed him to leave, but rather it was the subway death and the accumulation of years of secondary traumatization related to his health-care work that finally pushed him out. He is now working in his stepfather's business repairing residential home heating, ventilation, and air conditioning systems. Overall, he reports that he is much less stressed and has no intention of returning to the medical field.

## 4.2 Conceptualizations of Secondary Trauma in Health Professionals

There is an array of terms that are used in the professional literature to describe the transmission of distress from the sufferer to those who have a close connection to that person, such as a family member, close friend, or treatment provider, although this form of emotional contagion is not new. Jung (1966), for example, conceived of the notion of "unconscious infection" that can impact the therapist who is working with those experiencing various psychological disturbances. At times, selected secondary trauma terms are used when they describe reactions to the distress of family members, health-care professionals, those working with people with handicapping conditions, those who treat physical trauma, those who teach children with serious handicapping conditions, and those who deal with psychological and developmental traumas. Thus, we encounter terms like vicarious trauma, compassion fatigue, secondary trauma, secondary traumatic stress (STS), burnout, and others. As stated in the introduction, there seems to be little empirical research that would support the reported differences in these terms, and for that reason secondary trauma or secondary traumatic stress is used in this book to cover all such transfers of distress and trauma.

McCann and Pearlman (1990) report that studies of secondary or vicarious trauma focused on working with difficult populations of various kinds and these early studies used the term *burnout* to detail the burdens on both educators and health-care providers. Burnout was described as cynicism, boredom, depression, growing insensitivity, and discouragement that eventuate from health-care work. Contributing factors in the development of burnout were said to be the emotional demands of always being empathic, professional isolation, and ambiguous success. High and perhaps unrealistic self-imposed expectations leave the overly burdened health-care provider with consequent feelings of inadequacy and incompetence and therefore even higher levels of burnout than they might have had if their expectations were more modest.

However, according to McCann and Pearlman, working with trauma survivors, as contrasted with working with those experiencing more general psychological problems, was reported to be particularly difficult "because the therapist is exposed to the emotionally shocking images of horror and suffering that are characteristic of serious trauma" (McCann & Pearlman, 1990, p. 134). For this reason, secondary traumatic stress and vicarious trauma were considered by these authors to be more suitable terms than burnout. In these cases the emotional exhaustion or compassion fatigue (Figley, 1995) that accompanies many forms of health-care support is compounded by the emotional impact of dealing with severe traumatic experiences, such as war, rape, torture, and brutal assault. But again, the various terms, such as burnout, vicarious trauma, and secondary trauma, all imply a form of emotional distress and exhaustion that is a consequence of both difficult and heavy caseloads. If the provider also has high standards for what they consider a successful outcome, or they place heavy professional demands on themselves, this increases the intensity of the difficulties that they will encounter.

Motta (2021) proposed that factors contributing to the development of PTSD and presumably STS or secondary traumatic stress are not only the experiencing of frightening and distressing events but, importantly, the inability to escape the distressing situation. When escape is possible, one experiences some degree of control over the trauma situation, and this lessens the level of fear and the traumatic emotional impact. This issue of being able to escape a potentially traumatic situation has relevance to health-care providers in that their commitment to their professions, their professional identity, and the determination to be of help to those they serve all act as a sort of constraint or limitation on their capacity for escape. Objectively it would seem that these health-care professionals can simply leave their practices, hospitals, or clinics, but this form of escape is not often realistic. Health professionals have made a commitment to their patients, to the facilities in which they work, and to themselves to be present and to provide help to those in need. These commitments and professional identities create a psychological barrier, a constraint, or perhaps a moral barrier that interferes with escape. The outcome of these barriers or professional commitments is that emergency medical personnel, to use but one example, experience high levels of secondary trauma (e.g., Roden-Foreman et al., 2017). These authors found that low resilience and a history of personal trauma were factors that contributed to vulnerability to becoming secondarily traumatized. Although emergency room clinicians and other health-care providers could theoretically escape their stressful job demands, their professional obligations constrain them. Just as in PTSD where an inability to escape contributes to the development of that disorder, the perceived inability to escape appears to be a factor that may contribute to the development of STS among health-care providers. In cases of PTSD, the barrier to escape may be external, such as the forced entrapment that might occur in a forcible rape. In STS the barriers are often self-imposed because of one's professional commitments and the demands created by deeply held professional identities that emphasize caring for others.

## 4.3 Consequences of Primary and Secondary Trauma

To better understand what happens emotionally, behaviorally, and cognitively to health-care providers when they develop secondary or vicarious trauma, a good starting point is to examine the consequences of primary trauma or PTSD because many of the diagnostic sequelae of primary trauma are what is transferred to the health-care worker. This section will address specific cognitive, behavioral, and emotional consequences of secondary traumatization and will also address an important topic that has not received sufficient attention in the literature and that is the alteration of one's self-view, that is, the self-changes that occur pre- and post-trauma and secondary trauma.

The American novelist, playwright, and author Gertrude Stein (1922) is reported to have famously stated, "A rose is a rose is a rose." The same could be said about traumatic experiences. Regardless of whether the trauma is due to war, rape, abuse, assault, natural disaster, physical and emotional disorder, and so on, a trauma is a trauma is a trauma. In general, trauma results in common behavioral manifestations such as avoidance and hyperarousal; emotional responses, especially anxiety and depression; and cognitive responses such as memory problems, difficulty in focusing attention, and the occurrence of disturbing and intrusive thoughts, beliefs, and perceptions. Importantly, trauma often triggers an alteration in one's self-view (Motta, 2020, p. 20). The alteration is often in the direction of increased feelings of vulnerability and decreases in perceptions of self-worth, and these occur when one sees that they can no longer cope with a given traumatic situation. Previously, the now traumatized individual may have seen themselves as competent and capable of handling various difficult situations. Following overwhelming trauma, they now see themselves as far less capable and significantly more vulnerable.

These self-alterations are also experienced by health-care providers as they unwittingly begin to incorporate elements of their clients' trauma into their own lives. Providers may begin to see themselves as increasingly vulnerable and unable to cope. This was likely what took place in the health-care providers mentioned above who had to deal with the emotional and physical stressors of their patients and had to manage their own stressors by perhaps fantasizing about leaving their jobs, leaving their commitments, or committing suicide. Their identities were deeply tied to their roles as health-care professionals who were strong and able to support and guide patients through the worst of their suffering. Having become overwhelmed by a constant stream of distressed patients, these health-care providers could no longer cope. The limits of their capabilities had been exceeded. They became demoralized and probably wondered whether they were indeed cut out for the profession they had chosen.

Pearlman and Saakvitne (1995, p. 158) note that cynicism is a defining characteristic of secondary traumatization, and this negativistic attitude can permeate the organizations in which the health-care provider works in addition to negatively impacting one's sense of self. Other disturbing consequences of secondary trauma are reported by these authors to be disillusionment, despair, negativism, depression, and a decreased sensitivity and responsiveness to patient needs. Given the comorbidity of depression and anxiety (e.g., Gaspersz et al., 2018), it is not surprising that secondarily traumatized therapists who find themselves depressed may have a generalized and pervasive sense of anxiety along with apprehensions that are directly related to the client's problems, whether they be rape, childhood sexual abuse, or another traumatic event.

So, to summarize, those health-care providers experiencing secondary trauma have been altered emotionally, behaviorally, and cognitively. They find themselves to be anxious and depressed, avoidant, suspicious, and distrustful and have difficulties with concentration and memory. Their very view of themselves has been altered such that their prior self-view as a committed health-care professional is now replaced by a less sanguine and more cynical view of themselves, others, and their environments. These negative alterations are exacerbated by such factors as heavy trauma caseloads, prior difficulties encountered in their own childhoods, lower levels of resilience, and high expectations of themselves as health professionals. While not all these behavioral, emotional, and cognitive consequences are always present in secondary traumatization, many of them do in fact take place.

## 4.4 Case Example: The Trauma Psychotherapist

I discussed the case of Jordan in the previous chapter. Jordan is a COVID long hauler whose specific symptoms include persistent and long-running panic attacks, an intense claustrophobia involving the perception of his brain trapped inside of his skull, and physical issues such as debilitating fatigue and breathing difficulties. I have been the therapist involved in this case and have also worked with his family who are extremely secondarily traumatized by his frantic behaviors. He has attacked them physically while thrashing about in a panic attack, threatened suicide, made suicidal gestures, blamed them for his problems, and yet frantically begged them for help. He calls them and in a state of sobbing despair makes comments like "I can't live like this anymore," "My life is over," "This is the last time you will be hearing from me," and "I'm never going to get better; this is the end of me." These tearfully and frantically delivered calls initially occurred daily and continued for almost 6 months. After over a year of long-haul symptoms, Jordan began making progress in that he had a few days during the week when he could go to the gym, swim, and meet with friends at a coffee shop. However, he continued to be too impaired to resume his adjunct professor teaching activities. There were many days when he felt so frightened and overwhelmed that he could not get out of bed. And then, after his seeming progress, he again relapsed and had to be confined to different psychiatric and skilled nursing facilities.

I had seen Jordan on and off for years, prior to his COVID exposure, and helped him with problems such as mild anxiety, depression, and doubts related to his professional identity. In addition to my work as a trauma therapist, I also run a university-based general trauma clinic and am a full-time psychology professor. Despite having treated and supervised numerous and varied trauma cases, some of which involved intense suffering (Motta, 2021), I had never seen a more demanding and emotionally exhausting case than that presented by Jordan and his family. There have been weeks when I would receive almost daily calls from either Jordan, his mother, sister, or all three. His sister in particular calls or texts almost every day frantically seeking support. His family has been desperate to get help for Jordan, and his frantic suicide threats have resulted in multiple hospitalizations at different psychiatric facilities. In addition to trying to assist his family and provide them with emotional support, I found myself consulting with psychiatrists and other physicians involved in his care so that I could be better able to treat him. One day, for example, he broke his foot while jumping off a stairwell in a parasuicidal attempt. The treating physician called me to better understand why Jordan was so irrational. Similar calls and consultations occur almost every week. Numerous health-care providers have been involved with Jordan including physical therapists, health aides, hospital administrators, other hospital personnel, and any of a multitude of others whom his family has brought in to help care for him.

This work with Jordan and his family has been emotionally draining, and the term "compassion fatigue" seems most appropriately applied here. His extreme long-hauler symptoms produced an elevated apprehension of the virus on my part, and I found myself often putting on a mask despite being fully vaccinated against the virus. After several months of working with Jordan and his family, I found myself having nightmares about his potential to commit suicide. My clinic work and relatively heavy caseload added to the feeling of emotional exhaustion brought about by working with Jordan and his family. The case is ongoing and continues to produce a good deal of secondary traumatic stress and particularly feelings of emotional exhaustion. Working with Jordan and his family has been draining, but my professional commitment to him has tied me to his and his family's suffering.

There are several factors that have helped ameliorate the emotional burden presented by this case. My wife, a practicing psychologist, has been both supportive and helpful in providing suggestions for treatment. Professional colleagues have also been supportive and made specific intervention suggestions, although all admit that they have never dealt with a case as severe as this one. I make every effort to engage in forms of nontraditional intervention that have shown themselves to be helpful in dealing with traumatic stress including yoga, meditation, exercise, and immersion in nature. Specific interventions for secondary trauma will be discussed in later chapters. Another significantly helpful factor is the fact that Jordan, although continuing to be significantly psychologically impaired and unable to work, does occasionally show some signs that he is improving. His panic attacks are somewhat less intense and less frequent than they used to be, although he continues to have distressing episodes of panic and dissociation. He is showing glimmers of optimism, although admittedly these instances are few and far between. His family also appears to be better able to cope with Jordan's continuing challenges, and although I receive fewer frantic calls from them, the calls and texts continue at a high volume. In all, this case has given me a firsthand encounter with secondary traumatization. Jordan's mother, sister, and I have been on something of an emotional rollercoaster, but happily this jarring ride is beginning to become less wrenching as slow and continuing progress is being made. Compassion fatigue and secondary trauma are real and are a common outcome of working with traumatized individuals. It is important for health-care providers to know their own limitations and to try to lessen their emotional burdens when they begin to become overwhelmed. At this stage, I would probably not take on another COVID long-hauler case who was confronting wrenching negative emotional experiences as I, like all other practitioners, have limits to my emotional reserves.

## 4.5 Summary

While family members may be the most common sufferers of secondary traumatic stress, mental and physical health-care providers often encounter secondary trauma because of their work with those in distress. The symptoms of secondary trauma among health-care providers reflect many of the symptoms seen in the primary trauma and PTSD in those they treat. The symptoms of secondary trauma in health-care providers include anxiety, depression, emotional exhaustion, cynicism, demoralization, a negative alteration of their sense of self as a professional, and other related symptoms. The difficulties in shouldering the burdens of secondary trauma have led health professionals to a variety of treatment approaches, to leaving the field and, in a few disturbing cases, to taking their own life. Immediate interventions aimed at alleviating secondary trauma in treating professionals are sorely needed, and at the very least, a reduction in caseload may be an essential starting point. Secondary trauma among health-care providers is a serious matter and specific forms of intervention will be taken up in later chapters.

# Chapter 5
# Secondary Trauma in First Responders and Those Not Providing Professional Care

Prior chapters have dealt with secondary traumatization among professional health-care providers such as psychotherapists or medical personnel and with child and adult family members who often care for ailing or otherwise traumatized individuals. The secondary trauma that was produced among health-care providers and family members appeared to be principally related to the emotional depletion such as is seen in compassion fatigue (Figley, 1995) or the negative impact of emotional contagion (Hatfield et al., 1994) that these helpers acquired because of their work. However, the spread of trauma reactions has been documented in a surprisingly wide array of other samples of those who are not engaged in family caregiving or in direct therapeutic work (e.g., Figley & Ludik, 2017). This group includes, but is not limited to, firefighters, police officers, EMTs, lawyers, emergency room staff, librarians who deal with trauma-related inquiries and provide trauma-related material, taxi drivers, hairdressers, spouses of military combatants and first responders, insurance claims adjusters, judges, 911 dispatchers, pararescue personnel, suicide hotline responders, and many others. Ludick (2013), for example, found that 20% of insurance claims adjusters, a group one would not usually associate with secondary trauma, expressed emotional distress and secondary trauma symptoms owing to the frequency with which they had to deal with disturbing cases. Their levels of distress were not unlike that which is commonly seen in professional health service providers and military combatants. It appears that having a large and highly traumatized caseload, or many exposures to the trauma of others, affects these adjusters just as it does professional health-care specialists. Baird and Kracen (2006) have tied frequency of exposure to disturbing cases as an important factor in the development of STS. This appears to occur regardless of the nature of one's occupation if that occupation entails trauma exposure. Another important factor in the development of secondary trauma is the intensity of the pain experienced by the person who was primarily traumatized. Their level of emotional pain is felt proportionately among those who have close contact with that person (e.g., Suozzi & Motta, 2004). Sometimes the pain and terror experienced by the person who was directly

© The Author(s), under exclusive license to Springer Nature Switzerland AG 2023

R. W. Motta, *Secondary Trauma*, https://doi.org/10.1007/978-3-031-44308-4_5

traumatized ultimately leads to that person's death, whether by natural causes or suicide. The impact of the death produces secondary trauma reactions in first responders and in body handlers who are called on to remove remains.

Taylor and Fraser (1982) collected data on workers who were involved in the aftermath of the crash of a DC-10 airliner. In their sample of 180 such workers, high levels of emotional turmoil were found on standardized measures as were consequent health problems such as sleeplessness, loss of appetite, and increased social isolation. These symptoms were especially noted among body handlers. Beaton and Murphy (1993) surveyed two thousand Washington state paramedics and firefighters. They found that 80% of their sample reported anxieties related to their work and fears related to the vulnerability of themselves and their families. These two studies and those noted above, for example, Ludick (2013), highlight two important points. First, there is a large and varied group of professions that are involved in helping or managing others in a way that is not related to directly providing care. Even though they are not directly providing care, they are nevertheless vulnerable to developing secondary trauma. Second, there are differences in the nature and intensity of the trauma stimuli experienced by the various groups. Those involved in body recovery, such as in the Taylor and Fraser (1982) study, experience distressing events of a nature that differs markedly from that of insurance claims adjusters (Ludick, 2013). What these groups have in common is that they are exposed to distressing experiences even though they are not providing the direct care as are psychotherapists, nurses, and physicians. What they also have in common is that they are negatively impacted by the trauma that has impacted others. The group that is frequently addressed in the literature, especially regarding the unique and intense stressors they endure, is generically known as first responders. Their jobs are necessary to assure public safety but are also highly stressful.

## 5.1 Secondary Trauma in First Responders

Greinacher et al. (2019), in a systematic review of studies of secondary traumatization, identified first responders as police officers, firefighters, search and rescue personnel, or emergency and paramedic team members. Benedek et al. (2007) also included these professions in their definition of first responders, but the term *first responder* is somewhat arbitrary and might include other groups such as nonmedical ER personnel or even self-identified volunteer citizen groups composed of former first responders. One of the unifying risk factors encountered by first responders is the repetitive pace of their work. They appear to move quickly from one crisis to the next and as a result have little time to process and integrate their work experiences. Bentley et al. (2013), in a study of emergency medical service (EMS) personnel, found that 69% did not have time to recover from distressing events before being put upon to deal with additional potentially traumatic assignments and encounters. This unrelenting pace resulted in elevations of depression and trauma symptoms, such as intrusive cognitions, and suicidal ideation. Garbern et al. (2016)

found significant levels of clinical depression in over 21% of first responders to an earthquake in East Japan. EMS personnel reported higher peritraumatic stress symptoms such as dissociation at the time of the Loma Prieta Bay Area, San Francisco, California, earthquake (1989) in comparison to police officers (Marmar et al., 2006). Existing research suggests that EMS personnel have a lifetime prevalence of suicidal ideation and belief that life is not worth living that is significantly higher than the general population (Marmar et al., 2006).

However, even in the seemingly homogenous group of first responders, there appear to be important differences in the types of stressors they encounter. For example, police officers are not typically involved with burn victims as are firefighters, yet both groups encounter the suffering of others. Another of the many differences between these groups is that police officers, unlike firefighters, have had to deal with increasing public and political pressure and scrutiny over the involvement of some of their membership in the alleged violation of the rights of others, particularly those groups representing diversity. So, even though first responders appear to represent an identifiable cohort, the unique stressors they endure and the emotional consequences they experience can differ among their various groups.

There are even differences within groups of first responders. Stanley et al. (2017) found that career firefighters reported higher levels of problematic alcohol use and PTSD as compared to volunteer firefighters, while volunteers had higher levels of depression, suicidal ideation, and suicide attempts. The higher level of affective disorders among volunteers may have been due to the limited availability of mental health services for that group. Binge drinking was reported in 39.5% of the female firefighter population and 50% of male firefighters. Binge drinking in the general population is approximately 12–15% (Haddock et al., 2017). The common element among and within the various groups of helpers noted above appears to be the feeling of being overwhelmed and emotionally depleted by the suffering of others. It is difficult to say that any one group suffers greater or lesser levels of STS than any other group, but there are job and personal elements within and between groups that may make STS more or less likely.

For example, although there are few systematic studies regarding predisposing factors that would make one vulnerable to developing STS, some that have been noted are premorbid psychological adjustment, presence or absence of social support, quality of supervision within organizational settings, frequency, intensity of exposure to traumatic situations, personal history of abuse, and community support (Garbern et al., 2016). In this latter category of community support, we see police officers getting a mixed response from the community given some high-profile cases where they have mismanaged conflict situations. Their job demands and decreased levels of community support have led some authors to view police officers as being weighed down by trauma to the same degree as Vietnam War veterans (e.g., McCafferty et al., 1990) and as suffering from "demoralization and brutalization" (p. 546). It has also been suggested that the ongoing stressors of police work may result in impairments in judgment and executive functioning and that these difficulties may have led to reports of socially unacceptable behaviors on their part (Campbell, 2021). The demoralization of police officers could be due to unfair generalizations in which the problem behaviors of individual officers are also attributed to those whose who have not displayed socially troublesome behavior. The concept of "guilt by association" is apropos here in that the negative social impact occasioned by the problem behavior of the few spreads to the many. One of several high-profile cases that eroded community support and significantly added to police demoralization is that of Sandra Bland.

## 5.2 Case Presentation: Sandra Bland

History.com Editors (2020) reported a case that had a significant and widely reported negative impact on police officers and the community. Regrettably, the case is not unique. In 2015 a Texas state trooper, Brian Encinia, pulled over a car for failure to signal while changing lanes. The driver of the car was a Black 28-year-old female, Sandra Bland. After being pulled over, a heated exchange took place over Sandra's refusal to put out a cigarette and refusal to get out of her car, all of which was recorded by the trooper's dashcam. From her perspective she might have felt unfairly singled out and picked on because she was Black and perceived the traffic stop as an injustice that was difficult to tolerate. From the officer's viewpoint, she may have been disrespectful and defiant. The officer threatened her with his Taser and stated that he would "light her up" if she did not comply with his demands. At this point Bland got out of her car and a scuffle developed. Bland was knocked to the ground. Encinia claimed that Bland tried to kick him, and this is what resulted in the physical altercation, although kicking was not recorded on the dashcam video. Bland was taken to jail, and several days later when an officer tried to deliver her breakfast, she was found dead in her jail cell. She reportedly hung herself with a plastic garbage bag. Bland's family and friends protested her treatment by the police and raised questions over whether her death was due to suicide. The family stated that she had been in good spirits the day of her arrest and was enthusiastic about the start of a new job that was going to begin in a few days. Questions were also raised regarding whether protocol was followed in conducting prisoner observation while Bland was in jail. A media frenzy developed over this case, coming as it did a year after another high-profile case involving the death of a Black man, Eric Garner, at the hands of the New York Police Department, following his being placed in a prohibited chokehold. The position of the media was that these cases appeared to fit a pattern of police violence and targeted racism. The Bland and Garner cases fomented international outrage over police officer killings of Black citizens and became a rallying cry of the Black Lives Matter movement. Another incident in 2020 involving another Black man, George Floyd, who was arrested over a reputed attempt to pass a counterfeit 20-dollar bill resulted in a murder conviction of Officer Derek Chauvin who placed his knee on Floyd's neck and back for approximately 9 min and suffocated him. Video from bystander cell phones recorded Floyd stating "I can't breathe" several times. Chauvin did not respond to these pleas and continued impassively kneeling on Mr. Floyd until he was dead.

It is most unfortunate that cases such as those above are in no way isolated incidents and have reflected poorly on police departments, even to the extent of calls to "defund" the police. The relevance of these publicly reported instances of inappropriate behavior on the part of some police officers is that they add significantly to the already considerable stressors and secondary trauma experienced in police work. There has been an erosion of social and community support for police officers given the above situations and similar unfortunate incidents involving minority groups. Social support is one of the factors which, when in place, helps to mitigate the impact stressors on first responders (Beaton & Murphy, 1993), and it is this social and community support that is being taken away from police departments owing to the egregious behavior of a few of its members.

## 5.3 Forward Panic: An Extreme Reaction to Police Stressors

Police officers are frequently called upon to deal with problems such as traffic violations, family disputes, robberies, assaults, drug busts, shootings, and similar community difficulties. At times they must deal with armed assailants, and this is a particularly threatening and anxiety-provoking situation that can lead to a phenomenon known as "forward panic" (Collins, 2008). Forward panic is a sociological phenomenon that occurs when there is a conflict situation that exists between groups or individuals. Fear of the other group can result in an excessive and often violent overreaction that is substantially more than what is needed to resolve the conflict situation. Forward panic events, when publicized, can produce intense criticism from the community.

Such a case involving police officers and forward panic is fully detailed in Motta (2021, pp. 265–282). In this case, a seemingly schizophrenic individual was brandishing a shotgun and threatening his neighbors because he believed that they were demons in the disguise of humans. The police were called, and seven squad cars arrived on the scene. Neither the police nor the neighbors knew that the shotgun was not loaded. The police demanded that the individual put down the rifle, but he refused to do so and pointed it in their direction. Suddenly gunfire erupted and the man was shot to death. What was shocking in this encounter was the excessive overreaction of the police officers. They fired over one hundred rounds, and this was entirely unnecessary as the man in question was said to have been felled by the initially fired bullets. Many rounds impacted a seemingly lifeless body. Stray rounds hit neighboring homes and in one case nearly killed a teen watching television at home. This excessive response on the part of the police appears to have been due to the fear resulting from being confronted by an armed and seemingly dangerous individual who refused to respond to an order to put down his weapon. The neighbors were shocked by the overreaction by the police, and the local press also seemed to have no explanation for what happened. It appears that forward panic is the likely explanation for the police response, but again, just as in the Bland and other cases noted above, the image of the police and support from within the community was seriously tarnished. The resulting stain on the police department added to the stress inherent in police work, which in and of itself is sufficient to produce secondary trauma reactions. Such a negative community response and withdrawal of support are seldom seen for other groups of first responders such as firefighters, EMT personnel, and paramedics. In fact, these groups are often held in high regard and receive considerable levels of community support.

## 5.4 Psychological and Physiological Reactions in Secondary Trauma

Beaton and Murphy (1995) report several health consequences among those who are secondarily traumatized while engaging in community or first responder work. Exposure to the severely distressed, injured, or dead negatively impacts sleep puts stress on relationships, increases anxiety and a sense of dread, and produces depersonalization and derealization, which is the feeling that encountered situations seem unreal or hard to integrate with common experience. Also reported are nightmares, numbing of responsiveness, intrusive thoughts, and substance abuse. Physiological consequences include an increased rate of duodenal ulcers, pulmonary embolisms, cirrhosis of the liver, and infarctions at almost twice as high as rates in the general population (Beaton & Murphy, 1995, p. 60).

The fact that many crisis workers and first responders are imbued with the "John Wayne syndrome" (Mitchell, 1983) does not help matters. This identity mandates that they "should" be able to handle the stresses of their jobs. The macho self-view unfortunately results in many not seeking clearly needed support and assistance. This self-image is seen to a far lesser extent among other groups such as the insurance claim adjusters mentioned earlier, or the judges, dispatchers, and others not involved in first responder roles and these non-first responders may be more likely to seek help when they need it because they don't have a "tough guy" image that they must maintain.

A factor that appears to mitigate secondary traumatization, at least among first responders, has to do with the fact that these crisis workers have chosen their profession with full knowledge of the threats and dangers involved. To some extent they are drawn to the excitement and challenge of being on the front lines. As a result, the majority are not secondarily traumatized to an excessive degree (e.g., Hytten & Hasle, 1989). In a study of first responders that included police officers, firefighters, and paramedics who were involved in the aftermath of the World Trade Center attack in Manhattan, it was found that this group experienced moderate, but not severe, levels of trauma and secondary traumatization (Sciancalepore & Motta, 2004) on standardized measures and this was attributed to their training, preparedness, and professionalism. Again, their moderate, rather than severe, levels of secondary traumatization may have been because these first responders chose their profession and as a result were somewhat emotionally armed against being traumatized. Sciancalepore et al. also found that first responders' ability to cope with severe stressors was something that many wore proudly and that it often served as a vehicle for unit cohesion. Despite this, their levels of distress and secondary traumatization were found to be significantly higher than that which is seen in the general population.

One of the problems in conducting research that attempts to assess distress tolerance among self-selected groups such as first responders is that they may be subject to social desirability responding, that is, the tendency to not present themselves as vulnerable because this is not the socially expected norm for their group. As a result, there is a tendency to alter their responses on questionnaires to be in accord with traditional norms and expectations for their cohort. Another issue that might impact honest responses on research questionnaires is that the participants' self-expressed needs for health services, especially those involving psychological problems, can have negative consequences as far as career advancement is concerned. This is a problem often seen among military combatants (e.g., Motta, 2021) and perhaps uniformed first responders in general who are aware that seeking psychological services may be interpreted as weakness and negatively impact one's professional advancement. Another factor that decreases the accuracy of self-reports of psychological problems is that such admission of problems is in direct conflict with their own self-image of self-reliance and internal strength. A study by Greinacher et al. (2019) that collated data from over 30 scientific investigations found relatively low levels of secondary traumatization in first responders. It was suggested in this study that social desirability and job loss concerns may have contributed to the relatively low levels of measured secondary trauma and therefore secondary traumatization may have been higher than shown in the included studies. The authors do note, however, that resilience and social or community support for the important work that the first responders do might also be factors that mitigate the reporting of secondary trauma symptoms.

Beckman (2015) collected data on secondary traumatization experiences from 92 American Red Cross personnel who had responded to a national disaster within the prior 5 years. Among the risk factors of secondary traumatic stress were recent participation in a disaster response situation, being a young adult, and being single. Protective factors that decrease the chance of developing secondary traumatic stress were working with trauma survivors outside of their volunteer work and sometimes or always being engaged in self-care. It is assumed that being engaged in self-care serves to ameliorate the stressors involved in disaster work and creates a break from frequent and continuous exposure to traumatic situations. Like the study by Sciancalepore and Motta (2004) that investigated first responders in the World Trade Center terrorist attack, it was found that most participants did not develop significant symptoms of secondary trauma, although importantly 25% did in fact show some STS. This 25% figure is not insubstantial and is a significant mental health concern. However, the fact that the Red Cross participants had volunteered for disaster work suggests that they may have been somewhat armed against a high level of secondary trauma vulnerability because they expected to encounter such situations.

## 5.5 Risk and Protective Factors for Secondary Trauma in First Responders

There are many experiences that have been found to increase the chances of developing trauma-related difficulties due to being in direct contact with those who have been psychologically or physically impacted by negative experiences or who have lost their lives. Among the risk factors that increase the probability of developing secondary trauma among first responders are inadequate training, excessive and unrealistic expectations from supervisors, personal history of trauma and loss prior to engaging in trauma-related work, lack of community support as noted above, long hours, demanding circumstances, number of assignments, poor premorbid adjustment, and substance abuse (Brooks et al., 2016; Mitchell, 2011). Other factors that increase the chances of developing secondary trauma are not having time off, working in unfamiliar and demanding circumstances, fatigue, job dissatisfaction, dealing with the seriously injured or with dead bodies, excessive exposure to gory sights, working with injured children, low perceived safety, and having conflicting job demands (Brooks et al., 2015). Personal and personality factors associated with increased risk of developing STS include being overly sensitive, being introverted, having a generalized anxiety disorder, having family or marital problems, and feeling that one has not received acknowledgment or thanks for the risky and stressful work that first responders do. Avoidance coping, having specific fears, being neurotic, being introverted, and tending to avoid traumatic thoughts are all associated with increases in distress as seen in STS and an increase in PTSD (Brooks et al., 2015; Garbern et al., 2016; Waters, 2018).

In comparison to the numerous factors that contribute to the development of STS, there are fewer that serve to protect first responders. Among the protective factors that lessen the possibility of developing STS are quality of preparedness training, specialized training and assurance of personal and team mastery, and resilience (Brooks et al., 2015, 2016; Bryant, 2021; Haglund et al., 2007). Also found to be protective against STS were social and community support and organizational support, including good relationships with those in charge (e.g., Bryant, 2021). Organizational strategies that help in reducing STS are having clear protocols and strategies in place prior to the occurrence of specific crisis situations. This form of preparedness has been associated with better coping capabilities (Mitchell, 2011). Teamwork and a shared sense of community cohesiveness among first responders are also beneficial in strengthening one's capability to deal with traumatic situations (Quevillon et al., 2016). Personality factors such as being open, social, and extroverted have also been linked with better coping skills, perhaps because these characteristics can result in greater access to social support (Waters, 2018).

The issue of community cohesiveness (Quevillon et al., 2016) as a protective factor in mitigating the impact of STS is particularly relevant to those serving in police departments. According to an NPR (2021) news report, police departments have been receiving increased criticism from the community owing to having been accused of ethnic profiling and systemic racism. NPR reports on a 2021 survey of over 200 police departments that shows a 45% increase in retirement rates and a 20% increase in resignations. The survey was conducted by an organization called the Police Executive Research Forum, which suggested that a combination of low morale within the departments and scrutiny resulting from the negative press of high-profile cases, particularly involving Black citizens, was a leading cause of the retirements and resignations. The work of police officers and other first responders is psychologically demanding, and, in general, first responders cope well with the stressors inherent in their regular work. But, without the perception that their work is both valued and supported and with the ongoing concern that they may have to be looking over their shoulders for fear of being critiqued, the job becomes more difficult.

It has been suggested (Terill & Reisig, 2003) that law enforcement officers are part of, and reflect the values of, an institutional culture that sets the tone as to what is or is not permissible. This suggests that excessive force, especially against those representing minority groups, is tolerated and sometimes encouraged by those in command of the officers and that unless there is a change in the command culture, the problems within police departments will continue. From the point of view of the police officer, they are following administrative expectations and expect to be praised rather than vilified for their efforts. The fact that they receive criticism from the community in their attempts to do their job well makes the stressors of the job more difficult to tolerate.

## 5.6 Possible Benefits of Secondary Traumatization

When one reads the literature on trauma, secondary trauma, and PTSD, the usual emphasis is on the negative emotional, physical, and maybe even spiritual aspects of having been traumatized, but are there possible benefits? The purpose of this book is to elucidate the concept of secondary trauma with a particular emphasis on its negative consequences, just as the literature on PTSD focuses primarily on the impairments caused by this disorder. Unlikely as it may seem, there may be enhancing aspects that have been associated with both PTSD and STS. The German philosopher Friedrich Nietzsche is associated with variations of an 1888 quote, "Out of life's school of war – What does not kill me makes me stronger." Similarly, Calhoun and Tedeschi (2013, p. 6) cite an African proverb that "Smooth seas do not make skillful sailors." So, perhaps there is a positive side to the experience of distressful or traumatizing events in that they may strengthen one. Tedeschi and Calhoun (1996, 2004) are associated with the concept of posttraumatic growth, which is seen as an increased appreciation for life and an enhanced depth and perspective that can develop following traumatic situations. Thus, those who experience secondary traumatization may learn to better appreciate what they have, value the role they play in helping others, and generally be more content with themselves.

What are some of these positive effects? Those caring for family members who are ill or in the process of dying may feel that they have risen to, or are called to, an honored position of being entrusted with the care of a loved one. The fact that the caregiver can provide some level of relief to the sufferer can result in feelings of fulfillment and an increased sense of self-regard. A similar situation can occur among professionals such as mental health therapists, physicians, and nurses. Although they may be highly distressed and fatigued by the work they do and may suffer anxiety, depression, sleeplessness, and maybe even flashbacks, they derive a sense of purpose, fulfillment, and pride over being in a position where they can alleviate the psychological or physical distress of those whom they care for.

First responders, although not as personally involved as family members or direct care providers, experience a sense of satisfaction over having either saved a life or alleviated the distress of those who are traumatized. Oddly, these examples of posttraumatic growth are not considered to be the antithesis of secondary trauma or PTSD. It is not the case that the experience of growth vitiates or neutralizes the negative impact of trauma. Rather it appears that posttraumatic growth and trauma experiences, whether primary or secondary, can occur simultaneously. The clinician or first responder often experiences both distress and growth (Calhoun & Tedeschi, 2013). The suffering endured by family members, professional care providers, and first responders often induces a state of questioning the meaning of one's existence. Frankl (1963) suggests that suffering and the quest for meaning that often follows suffering can result in a deeper and more aware sense of self. None of this is meant to minimize the long and often intense suffering that is associated with secondary traumatization but rather is presented to give a fuller picture of what is entailed in the experience of having been secondarily traumatized.

## 5.7 Summary and Thoughts on Intervention

First responders and others who are not involved with the direct care of family members can nevertheless experience secondary traumatization. There is a wide array of such helpers, but this group typically involves firefighters, EMTs, paramedics, disaster responders, and police officers, among others. This chapter highlights factors that increase the probability of these groups developing secondary trauma including long working hours, moving from one crisis to the next, lack of administrative support, lack of training, and other factors. A particular emphasis on the role of lack of community support especially as experienced by some police departments was highlighted as contributing significantly to secondary trauma. The lack of community support was tied to resignations, retirements, and demoralization. Protective factors that lower the probability of secondary trauma were quality of training, group cohesiveness, being outgoing and socially engaged, and having available support services as well as social and community support. Although secondary traumatic experiences can be both draining and exhausting, the positive side of this disorder, called posttraumatic growth, was also presented. Posttraumatic growth does not negate or neutralize secondary trauma but rather frequently occurs along with it. Posttraumatic growth is often associated with a deepening of perspective, increased sensitivity to the needs of others, and an enhancement of one's self-perception.

Those within families who care for a sick or traumatized member, those who provide direct psychotherapeutic or medical care, and those who function in the capacity of first responders are all impacted differently and yet similarly can develop secondary trauma symptoms. Family members represent the largest group of those who experience secondary trauma, and it might be argued that given the intense bonds that can exist within families, they may be the most severely impacted. Watching a family member suffer from a painful and progressive illness such as might be seen in terminal cancer is an emotionally wrenching and exhausting experience. Days can be consumed with intense worry and fatigue and nights that produce rest-destroying nightmares and sleeplessness. Many in these situations, despite the intensity of their "compassion fatigue," feel compelled to stay with the distressed family member out of love and a compelling desire to alleviate suffering. The exhaustion, anxiety, and depression are all a heavy price to pay, but family members simply cannot walk away from the need to provide care.

It has been well documented that therapists also pay a heavy emotional price for the care they provide to their traumatized clients (e.g., McCann & Pearlman, 1990). The emotional drain in working with some of their more suffering clients can be considerable and can result in significant life disruptions. And while therapists are tied to their clients by their professional obligations and emotional connections, they appear to have more access to self-care than do family members. Therapists can engage in distracting and pleasurable activities as a way of ameliorating the burdens of their work. They can have consuming hobbies and other distracting activities that they can access to give themselves a break from the stresses of providing regular therapeutic assistance. In having these alternate, distracting activities available to them, they may endure a lesser, though still significant, level of secondary trauma than do family members.

First responders such as police officers, firefighters, EMTs, and paramedics are impacted by the sometimes shockingly disturbing situations they encounter and by the suffering they regularly see. However, in general, their emotional involvement is less than that of direct care providers or family members. Another factor that helps to ameliorate their stress is that they have chosen a line of work that they know will involve emergency situations and have been, in most instances, trained to deal with these situations. Their long hours, large number of crisis cases, and, in instances involving police departments, erosion of community support, all work to make their work emotionally distressing. First responders often have higher rates of substance abuse and higher rates of suicidal ideation and suicidal intention than the general population, all of which validate the fact that they are significantly impacted by secondary trauma that is inherent in being on the front lines when emergency services are needed.

## 5.8 Are There Interventions That Might Be Helpful for Secondary Trauma?

There is an emotional cost to caring for others regardless of whether that caring involves family members, clients and patients, or situations demanding urgent professional intervention. It is conventional to assert that this "compassion fatigue" is the price of being human, but it was shown earlier that animals can also show this concern. The literature on trauma and PTSD provides a good deal of empirically based information on many forms of therapeutic intervention that have been effective in treating this disorder. The zeitgeist driving the choice of intervention for PTSD falls heavily on the side of cognitive-behavioral types of intervention (e.g., Preston et al., 2002). In reviewing the literature on secondary traumatization, one finds no such unanimity of opinion regarding the appropriate therapeutic intervention. It is even reasonable to question whether therapeutic intervention is needed at all in most cases of secondary trauma. If there is an emotional cost to caring and such caring is a normal human activity, why is psychotherapy needed at all? It is to this issue to which we will now turn.

# Chapter 6
# Secondary Trauma Treatment Considerations

Prior chapters have described the origins and presentation of the emotional burdens of secondary traumatization in different populations. If we were to take the not universally accepted position that secondary traumatic stress is "a syndrome of symptoms that is nearly identical to PTSD …" (Figley, 1995, p. 8; Jenkins & Baird, 2002), then it would be logical to assume that the treatments for secondary trauma should also be "nearly identical" to that which have been used in the treatment of PTSD. Harris, 1995, states (p. 112), "In fact at present and in this author's experience, there is little, if any, difference between the treatment processes for PTSD and STSD" (secondary traumatic stress disorder). Similarly, Greinacher et al. (2019, p. 3) state, "More particularly, STS describes symptoms identical to PTSD …" If this view is valid, then we should know a good deal about treating STSD as there is a substantial literature on the treatment of PTSD, whether it involves the use of traditional treatments or nontraditional methods. However, this is not the case as there are few empirically supported studies to be found in the literature supporting specific treatments for secondary trauma or that compare the relative efficacy of specific treatments to others (Bercier & Maynard, 2015). None of this is meant to minimize the contributions of major contributors to the literature on secondary trauma such as Charles Figley and others, but there is a minimal knowledge base of empirical treatment efficacy studies of secondary trauma.

The zeitgeist for what might be seen as traditional and effective treatment for PTSD is cognitive-behavioral psychotherapy (CBT) (e.g., Foa et al., 2000; Preston et al., 2002). The basis of CBT is that dysfunctional and maladaptive thoughts are a primary cause of unwanted emotions and that the therapeutic correcting of these erroneous thoughts will reduce unpleasant feelings. CBT also emphasizes the development of helpful and adaptive behaviors to facilitate a healthier adjustment. Another approach used in CBT is exposure to and reliving of prior traumatic experiences through a process called "prolonged exposure" (e.g., Foa et al., 2007; Foa & Kozak, 1986). The goal in using prolonged exposure for treating PTSD is to reduce the negative psychological impact of traumatic events by repeated exposure to them rather than avoiding them and in this way becoming inured to their impact. In addition to the traditional treatment of CBT, there are nontraditional treatments.

© The Author(s), under exclusive license to Springer Nature Switzerland AG 2023

R. W. Motta, *Secondary Trauma*, https://doi.org/10.1007/978-3-031-44308-4_6

Nontraditional treatments for PTSD include such distress-relieving approaches as yoga, meditation, exercise, engagement with nature, and other such interventions (Benedek & Wynn, 2016; Motta, 2021). Their value in treating PTSD is that they are easier to tolerate than the psychologically confronting approaches that are used in CBT involving the reexperiencing of traumatic events and the challenging of thoughts that are considered dysfunctional. These nontraditional approaches to treating secondary trauma are not based on the foundational position of CBT, namely, that dysfunctional thoughts are the cause of emotional distress. Rather, the nontraditional approaches are specifically aimed at alleviating the distress directly, regardless of its cause. There are sound empirical studies that support the use of specific nontraditional treatments for PTSD, but these studies are not as abundant as those involving CBT (e.g., Gallegos et al., 2017; Hilton et al., 2017; Whitworth et al., 2017).

Despite the assertions of some authors (e.g., Harris, 1995) that PTSD and STSD treatments should be similar, what is found is that in comparison to the voluminous literature on the treatment of traumatic experiences and PTSD, the literature on the treatment of secondary trauma is both scant and fragmented and does not support the position of similarity of treatments for STSD and PTSD. There are virtually no psychometrically validated studies supporting the position that STSD and PTSD should be treated similarly. For example, a family member caring for another family member who has a progressively deteriorating illness is not necessarily suffering from dysfunctional thoughts that would warrant the use of CBT. It is possible that they are simply emotionally drained and saddened to see a loved one suffering. There is little in the way of irrational or dysfunctional thinking in this situation, and therefore the use of CBT, a common treatment for PTSD, would seem misguided. Typical dysfunctional thoughts seen in PTSD might include black-and-white thinking, overgeneralization, a tendency toward personalization, and others. Few, if any, of these cognitive errors appear to be involved in the distress of one family member caring for another. Relief from the distress in this situation might involve having others take over their caretaker duties, engaging in pleasurable distractions and hobbies, getting suitable exercise and rest, benefiting from social support of friends, and maybe even supportive counseling where the suffering family member can unburden themselves of their "compassion fatigue" (Figley, 1989; Norcross, 2000). There is not only little that is published about the efficacy of treatments of STSD, but there is even less in the way of controlled, data-based studies, especially those that compare treatments to each other. What do exist regarding the treatment of STSD are positions, views, and opinions put forth by those who have been involved in studying and treating STSD.

## 6.1 Family Caregivers

An example of a position statement regarding the treatment of secondary trauma is that of Figley and Kiser (2013) and Figley (1989) concerning intervention for distressed families. As noted earlier, families are the major source of the development of secondary traumatization. Figley reports that treatment of secondary trauma within families should include eight strategies. These are (1) building rapport and trust between therapist and family members; (2) clarifying the therapist's role; (3) eliminating unwanted consequences of traumatic experiences, such as discouragement and negativism; (4) building supportiveness among family members; (5) developing new roles and skills of family communication; (6) promoting self-disclosure; (7) recapitulating the traumatic events; and (8) building a family healing theory, and by this Figley (1989) is referring to "building a new and more optimistic perspective" (p. 65). This eight-stage approach appears to be based on the author's extensive treatment experience and abundant contributions to the literature on secondary trauma, but it does not seem to be empirically validated in any apparent way, nor can we find a comparison of this approach to other potential alternative treatments. Figley may be correct in suggesting that secondary traumatization often involves all members of the family, and for that reason he sees some form of family intervention as being necessary, but empirical support for this position by way of treatment comparison studies is lacking.

It may be the case that in certain instances of extremely distressful secondary traumatization within families, the lines between STSD and PTSD become blurred, and treatment approaches between these conditions may therefore be similar. One can conceptualize these two disorders as having some degree of overlap as might be seen in juxtaposed frequency distributions where the tail of one distribution overlaps the other. Another way of envisioning the possible overlap between PTSD and STSD that might occur in extremely distressing situations is to imagine these two stress disorders as a Venn diagram where some degree of melding between the two occurs. But in general, the two disorders appear to be distinct in that PTSD is typically caused by extreme threat and fear and STSD often eventuates from emotional exhaustion that develops from constantly giving of oneself in the service of others. The *DSM-5* (p. 271) states that PTSD can occur when there is "exposure to actual or threatened death, serious injury or sexual violence …" although "first responders collecting human remains …." could also develop PTSD. In other words, there are unique and extreme situations from which first responders might develop PTSD instead of STSD, but this is typically not the case. STSD is most often due to emotional exhaustion and "compassion fatigue" not from highly traumatizing experiences. If highly traumatizing experiences do occur, we are now within the diagnostic domain of PTSD and not that of STSD.

## 6.2 Professional and Paraprofessional Trauma Workers

Dutton and Rubenstein (1995) have described therapeutic interventions for trauma workers. By trauma workers these authors include those professionals and paraprofessionals who take remedial or restorative action in the aftermath of traumatic events. This group of trauma workers includes physicians, therapists, counselors, firefighters, paramedics, police officers, and others. The authors group interventions for secondary trauma into three areas: work-related strategies, informal strategies, and personal strategies. Among the work-related strategies are efforts to diversify one's caseload to reduce the emotional demands placed on the provider or paraprofessional. This might involve attempting to see fewer seriously impaired individuals and trying to engage in work-related behavior that is not involved with direct contact, for example, teaching, developing intervention strategies, and supervising others. Informal strategies involve engagement in consuming hobbies, maintaining social support networks, and spending time with family and friends. Personal strategies might entail seeking therapy to identify personal mediators that might make the worker more vulnerable to developing STSD. An example here might be the reactivation of a personal trauma history, which increases the worker's vulnerability to STSD. Another mediator might be having unrealistic expectations of the degree to which the worker feels they have to succeed in improving the plight of all the distressed individuals they encounter. But like the positions of Figley and Kiser (2013) and Figley (1989) regarding the need for family therapy, the treatment suggestions suggested by Dutton and Rubenstein (1995) have not been subject to thoughtful empirical evaluation.

## 6.3 Similarities and Differences Between PTSD and STSD

While there may be similarities between PTSD and STSD, the position that these two disorders are "nearly identical" (Figley, 1995) is questionable. Their similarity is that they both result in emotional distress that can persist and which often negatively influence one's general perspective on life and living. Their difference, in this writer's view, is that PTSD typically originates from an extreme fear, often a fear of life threat, and this is seldom the case with STSD. The negative emotional consequences of PTSD appear to be more severe than those of STSD (e.g., Adams et al., 2001; Suozzi & Motta, 2004; Wasco & Campbell, 2002). According to the *DSM-5* (American Psychological Association, 2013), PTSD can develop following exposure to threatened or actual death, assault, sexual violence, and similarly extremely frightening encounters. Contrast this with the secondary traumatization that occurs within families, which is a major source of the origin of STSD. Family members who develop secondary trauma are preoccupied with the suffering of a loved one and do everything in their power to reduce this distress. There is little of the intense fear that is typically found in the development of PTSD.

Similarly, the therapist, physician, firefighter, or paramedic suffering from STSD may become emotionally exhausted by the overwhelming demands inherent in their duties. In the case of secondary trauma, unlike PTSD, the source of distress arises from the provision of aid and the resulting emotional drain that eventuates from providing this succor and assistance especially to those who are seriously traumatized. In contrast, PTSD typically involves intense fear and a sense of disruptive vulnerability and, importantly, the felt inability to escape the threat (Motta, 2021, p. 8). Unlike STSD, PTSD is diagnosed by specific criteria as set forth by the *DSM-5* (2013), and these criteria are validated through empirical investigation. No such criteria or abundant sources of data-based research appear to be available for STSD. The point being made here is that while there are similarities between PTSD and STSD, their differences do not seem to warrant being seen as "nearly identical," nor is there suitable empirical justification for asserting, as does Harris (1995), that there should be little, if any difference, in the treatment of these two disorders. There is simply no empirical justification for taking that position.

As stated earlier, there are doubtlessly some extreme cases of STSD that might be indistinguishable from PTSD, but in general this appears to not be the case. The current writer has experienced PTSD due to having participated as a combatant in the Vietnam War (Figley also served in Vietnam) and has encountered secondary trauma due to his work as a trauma therapist and does not see these two disorders as in any way identical. In fact, their differences appear to outweigh their similarities by a wide margin. PTSD is a far more life-altering, self-perception changing, and environmentally fear-producing disorder than STSD.

Those who experience PTSD are often negatively transformed by this disorder, and this transformation can result in the phenomenological experience of being two people (van der Kolk, 2014). One person is the one that is seen in public: the teacher, accountant, and landscaper, for example. The other is a wary, suspicious, frightened entity whose behavior can often more resemble that of an unnerved animal than that of a human being. The person with PTSD has a negatively altered sense of self, and this is seldom seen in STSD. Those suffering from PTSD see themselves as having the undesirable characteristics of suspiciousness, distrust of others and of the environment, and a pronounced tendency toward isolation. The isolation appears to be due to the need to reduce feelings of vulnerability because they were threatened or harmed by environmental influences. As a result, they are now constantly on guard, hyperalert, and prone to overreact to perceived threats, which unfortunately seem to be everywhere. And while it is true that psychotherapists who are secondarily traumatized may share some of these characteristics, especially an alteration of prior beliefs regarding the predictability and safety of their environments (McCann & Pearlman, 1990), the magnitude of the change in one's perspectives and the degree of self-alteration appear to be far more profound and disabling in PTSD than in STSD. Similarly, family members of those who have PTSD can sometimes develop fears and aversions that are like those of the traumatized person, but these responses are seldom of the same magnitude as that of the PTSD sufferer. As van der Kolk (2014) asserts, the person suffering from PTSD is so deeply altered that they have a shadow self, a deeply wounded self, that they hide from the public.

This negative self-alteration and isolation often seen in PTSD are less apparent in secondary traumatization, and in fact, it is not unusual for helpers of various kinds to feel some degree of "compassion satisfaction" (Sprang et al., 2007) and self-enhancement in what they do, and not feel negatively altered (Stamm, 2010). For example (Eidelson et al., 2003), a survey study of the reactions of psychologists dealing with those who experienced the World Trade Center (WTC) terrorist attack found that therapists were confronted with clients who recounted terrible losses in graphic detail and that the closer therapists were to the WTC, the greater their experienced stress. Even though therapists in this survey often identified with the traumatic experience of their clients and the reality that this was a human-made and intended act, they nevertheless reported "a significantly greater increase in positive as opposed to negative feeling about their work" (p. 149). Secondary, or vicarious, trauma is doubtlessly a debilitating psychological problem, but it lacks the profound cognitive, emotional, behavioral, identity, and perhaps spiritual impairments commonly seen in PTSD. In a report on psychotherapists, Norcross (2000) reports that even though therapy can be an emotionally grueling profession, especially when dealing with traumatized clients, therapists often feel "enriched, nourished, and privileged in conducting psychotherapy" and that the work brings "joy, meaning, growth vitality, growth ..." despite the "strains of this 'impossible profession'" (p. 712). In contrast, although there is a possibility of posttraumatic growth (Calhoun & Tedeschi, 2013) following traumatic experiences, it seems unlikely that the person experiencing PTSD due to rape, combat, assault, sexual abuse, and other trauma would describe the outcome of their experience as resulting in feelings of being "enriched, nourished, and privileged ..." The equating of PTSD and STSD or secondary trauma simply seems unjustified.

## 6.4 What Are Effective Interventions for STSD?

It is unfortunate that therapists have little by way of empirical and/or controlled studies that would help them choose effective interventions for STSD. In addition, the source of secondary trauma may be an important issue that informs the type of treatment that might be initiated, and these sources vary. For example, those suffering from *family-related* secondary trauma might (or might not) benefit from family therapy as suggested by Figley (1989) and Figley and Kiser (2013) or might be relieved simply from relief or being "spelled" from the heavy caring burdens that they carry. Distracting activity and social support might also be helpful. *Professionals and paraprofessionals* who are burdened by repeated encounters with traumatized individuals might benefit from a reduction in caseload and participation in various forms of distraction (e.g., Bober & Regehr, 2006). They might also benefit from some form of intervention that targets their need to "rescue" all those who are presented to them for care. *Psychotherapists* might benefit from their own counseling and gain insight into their tendency to take on the dysfunctional perspectives of those whom they treat (McCann & Pearlman, 1990; Norcross, 2000). All these suggested interventions and the intentional use of the word "might" for the varied secondarily traumatized populations are well reasoned and based on a literature produced by those who have been involved in treatment and research on trauma and secondary trauma. However, they do not appear to be based on data-based and placebo-controlled studies for the most part. In fact, Bercier and Maynard's (2015) review shows that there are virtually no well-established guidelines for treating secondary trauma.

Among the few studies that investigated the effectiveness of interventions for secondary trauma in therapists was that of Bober and Regehr (2006). These authors found that secondary trauma was minimally impacted by individual initiatives such as self-care and distraction activities, and this finding appears to contradict the importance placed on self-care by some authors (e.g., Figley, 2002; Stamm, 2010). Rather, they found that hours per week spent working with traumatized people was correlated with secondary trauma development. They conclude that "it is perhaps time that vicarious and secondary trauma intervention efforts with therapists shift from education to advocacy for improved and safer working conditions" (Bober et al., p. 8). These findings lead to the conclusion that exposure reduction or reduction in the number of cases or engagements with those who have been traumatized or who have otherwise been severely distressed is one of the few validated ways of reducing secondary trauma. One cannot conclude from this study that exposure reduction is the only effective intervention, but it is one of the few interventions that have been supported empirically.

It is possible that other interventions might be of value, and while these might be worthy of consideration, there are distressingly few studies to support these. For example, it is possible that grief counseling, "rap" groups, nondirective counseling, engagement with nature or animals, or any number of other approaches could help alleviate the distress of secondary trauma. Clearly, further research is needed to address the question of efficacy of interventions for secondary trauma. The little research on the alleviation of secondary traumatization can be unfortunately contradictory. While Bober and Regehr (2006) found that reduction of trauma cases in one's caseload might be helpful in reducing secondary trauma, the opposite was reported in a recent study by Oginska-Bulik et al. (2021). These researchers found that job satisfaction, including having a large caseload, was associated with lower levels of secondary traumatic stress among medical professionals. Overall, however, the weight of evidence does seem to favor reduction of caseload, or leaving the field, as being associated with secondary trauma reductions (e.g., Bober & Regehr, 2006; Figley, 1995; van Dernoot Lipsky, 2009; Wright, 2016).

## 6.5 Summary and Proposed Presentation of Treatment Strategies

From the available literature, it appears that secondary traumatization and its putatively more severe variant, STSD, are caused by known sources. Some of these include providing support for suffering family members, the emotionally draining activity of providing therapy for cases impacted by trauma, repeated and demanding medical interventions, and the provision of community services of the kind associated with police officers, paramedics, search-and-rescue personnel, EMTs, and other groups. The emotional exhaustion, cynicism, and "compassion fatigue" that eventuates from these activities have been extensively documented in the literature. The intensity of this exhaustion, and at times demoralization, can become so extreme that it sometimes results in the care provider either leaving the field or taking their own life as noted in Chap. 4. Secondary traumatization is a serious problem that appears to result from being a caring individual. Sometimes this caring individual need not be human as empathic responding has been seen in primates (Chap. 1), and this concern for others can continue to the point where the aide provider's health and well-being are endangered.

While it is reported that PTSD and secondary traumatization are nearly identical (e.g., Figley, 1995; Jenkins & Baird, 2002), the position taken here is that their differences outweigh their similarities, although there can be clear overlap between the disorders (Bercier & Maynard, 2015; Suozzi & Motta, 2004). Regarding intervention, there is abundant literature on validated PTSD treatments, but in contrast, the data-based literature on secondary trauma treatment is scant. One empirically based study (Bober & Regehr, 2006) found that the usual self-care recommendations for those who might be secondarily traumatized were ineffective and that reducing individual demands on providers was helpful. However, no single study should be taken as validation for a given stance including this one. It is possible that there are intervention strategies that do alleviate secondary trauma and that the reduction in caseload as suggested by Bober et al. is not the only effective one.

The chapters to follow will focus on potentially effective interventions for secondary trauma. It appears that secondary traumatization is most often not caused primarily by dysfunctional thoughts that would then warrant CBT as a logical intervention, although this could be the case in unique circumstances. Rather, secondary trauma is seen as primarily, although not exclusively, due to the emotional drain and exhaustion eventuating from giving of oneself for the benefit of others. This giving can occur in many different contexts. The emotional drain and depletion can significantly impair one's functioning, and it would therefore appear that intervention strategies might best be oriented toward some form of alleviation of this distress.

Aside from reducing the emotional demands on the caregiver such as limiting caseloads or obtaining help in dealing with an ill family member, such common stress-relieving activities as exercise, controlled relaxation, meditation, yoga, natural environments, and other approaches will be described. It is important to restate that in most, but not all, circumstances, secondary trauma comes about because of emotional depletion following the helping, assisting, and caring for others and is rarely, if ever, due to life threat as in PTSD. Some of the alternative, non-CBT interventions that are presented have been shown to ameliorate the symptoms of PTSD and might be expected to be helpful in alleviating the distress of secondary trauma. For each intervention the attempt will be made to show how that intervention might be of value in treating secondary trauma due to the typical sources. These sources of secondary traumatization include that which arises due to family caregiving, to working as a professional therapist or medical provider, or to serving as a paraprofessional frontline worker. The chapter to follow on "structural interventions" will present general strategic methods of managing secondary trauma.

# Chapter 7
# Structural Interventions

The term *structural intervention* is being used here to distinguish these forms of dealing with secondary trauma from traditional individually administered therapeutic interventions such as CBT or any of the offshoots of CBT like acceptance and commitment therapy (ACT) (Hayes et al., 2016), dialectical behavior therapy (DBT) (Linehan, 1993), cognitive processing therapy (CPT) (Resick, 2001), and prolonged exposure (PE) (Foa & Kozak, 1986). Examples of structural interventions would include such activities as engaging the family in counseling or practical approaches such as reducing workload, improving quality of training, restructuring one's caseload, obtaining more training oriented toward managing specific kinds of traumatic occurrences, managing family stressors, improving supervision, engaging in various relaxation or meditative activities, and similar interventions that do not represent formal psychotherapy. Structural interventions focus primarily on changes in the work or family environment but also include specific stress-reducing activities, such as relaxation training, engagement in social activities, meditation, and yoga.

Some strengths of structural interventions are that they are practical, easy to understand, and relatively easy to implement. They are straightforward and are much unlike the bewilderingly complex flow diagrams and arcane explanations of secondary trauma and its treatment as exemplified in the graphical depictions and diagrams of some authors (e.g., Beaton & Murphy, 1995, p. 56; Remer & Ferguson, 1998, p. 153). Such complex representations of secondary trauma and its treatment might pique the interest of some academics but seem of little practical utility to those who experience and treat secondary trauma.

CBT and other forms of individualized psychotherapy might certainly be needed in cases and situations where one is required to perform body handling and retrieval, when one is attacked or had their life threatened while fulfilling their community job duties, when one is witness to horrific mutilation and death, or other extreme and shocking encounters. These intensely traumatic experiences might occur while one is engaging in activities such as search and rescue, participation in EMT or paramedic activities, fighting fires, doing police work, or performing medical or

© The Author(s), under exclusive license to Springer Nature Switzerland AG 2023

R. W. Motta, *Secondary Trauma*, https://doi.org/10.1007/978-3-031-44308-4_7

psychological interventions. However, as pointed out earlier, these experiences fall more into the category of events that are often associated with PTSD (*DSM-5, 2013)* and less so with secondary trauma. The former diagnosis is often the outcome of experiencing extreme fear and life threat, while the latter is associated with emotional depletion and exhaustion due to giving of oneself in the service of others. The position taken here is that emotional depletion, compassion fatigue, and similar emotionally demanding occurrences do not necessarily benefit from efforts to alter or reframe one's cognitions or to engage in repeated exposure to trauma stimuli as is done in CBT. Rather, practical, "non-therapy" forms of intervention are needed. Again, traditional forms of therapy may be needed when trauma exposure becomes intense, but not when the cause of distress is emotional depletion. So, what might these structural interventions look like?

## 7.1 Family Strategies

As was pointed out in the introduction and in Chap. 3, families are the major sources of secondary trauma in that a large percentage of families are coping with an impaired family member. The impairment of the family member could be due a physical illness, a psychological or emotional difficulty, a war experience, an assault, a serious automobile accident resulting in injury or death, or any number of other traumatizing experiences. In situations such as these, the individual's trauma spreads in a contagion-like fashion to the other member of the family and depletes them emotionally. Figley (e.g., 1989, Figley & Figley, 2009; Figley & Kiser, 2013) has been a driving force in popularizing concepts such as secondary trauma, compassion fatigue, and family interventions for burnout and secondary traumatization. He also served as a combatant in the Vietnam War, and despite his position on the similarity, or even sameness, of PTSD and secondary traumatization, they nevertheless clearly differ in both their origin and treatment.

Figley and Figley (2009, p. 181) states that "Most traumatologists continue to focus primarily on individuals and largely ignore families, the social support they provide and the mechanisms they develop for managing … consequences of traumatic events." Thus, his favored approach to dealing with secondary traumatization is to focus the intervention on the family. Figley and Figley (2009) suggests that when evaluating the efficacy of family treatment approaches for secondary trauma, the following six criteria are central:

1. Do no harm. Family therapy should assure safety and not expose family members to overly distressing traumatic memories. Safety for all members should be assured.
2. Exposure titration control. This criterion is considered one of the most important because it can help the client or family recall the traumatic memories and "modulate their reactivity to these memories" (p. 181). This criterion is like the method of prolonged exposure to trauma (PE) (Foa et al., 2007) but in a graded, easily tolerated, step-by-step form, so as not to be perceived as overwhelming.

3. Evidence of effectiveness. What is being suggested here is that there should be some way of assessing the outcome of the implemented interventions. For example, one might have pre- and post-assessments based on standardized trauma measures or even on ratings provided by members of the family.
4. Reciprocal inhibition tuning. One way the sympathetic nervous system (SNS) reacts to traumatic events is by the release of adrenaline and the engagement of a fight, flight, or freeze response. The "tuning" that Figley and Figley (2009) is addressing implies that it is helpful for traumatized individuals to engage in activation of the SNS but also to learn how to mute that response through parasympathetic activation (e.g., release of serotonin through relaxation exercises, laughter, and mindfulness). This modulation of the SNS is a learned and helpful skill for families and traumatized family members. What is essentially being learned here are coping skills for managing distress when it does occur.
5. Fit and fidelity. Fidelity refers here to the degree of accuracy that the applied intervention maintains in comparison to how it was initially designed and conceived (Holter et al., 2003). Fit refers to how well the therapist aligns the intervention with the needs and capabilities of the family. If the family is not able to tolerate a given intervention, it should be avoided regardless of the level of its empirical backing.
6. Quantity and quality of training. This criterion addresses the need for therapists to be well trained, to continue their training through such activities intermittent therapeutic learning activities, and to have access to quality supervision to further assure their competence in managing secondary trauma.

With the above general guidelines for structuring family interventions, Figley and Kiser (2013) discuss a five-phase approach to treating families impacted by trauma. These phases included in their "family empowerment therapy" include the following: joining the family, understanding and framing of treatment, building coping skills, sharing and healing, and moving forward. These phases essentially summarize those that were originally presented by Figley (1989) and are detailed below to show how secondary trauma within families is strategically managed.

## 7.2 Figley's Strategic Phases for Treating Secondary Trauma Within Families

Figley (1989) presents five treatment "phases" for dealing with what is typically a situation where the trauma of an individual has impacted the family and as a result has produced secondary traumatization within the family. In general, Figley focuses on the whole family as the primary target of treatment.

Phase 1. Building a commitment to therapeutic objectives. "The early phase of any systematic, professional intervention is primarily dedicated to building a sound therapeutic alliance between therapist and family clients" (Figley, 1989, p. 69). This, of course, is a meaningful way to begin any therapeutic interaction whether with individuals, groups, or families. During this phase there is an assessment of the family's traditional ways of coping, their resources, and how they individually conceive of and understand the nature of the trauma.

Phase 2. Framing the problem. The focus here is to elicit memories from each family member about the nature of the trauma, to provide rules of communication, to stay away from blame, and to shift attention from what happened or is happening to the traumatized individual to what is happening to the family.

Phase 3. Reframing the problem. In this phase the attempt is made to get the family to reach some degree of consensus about their views so that the problems become more manageable and tractable. It is important here not to rush the process. The family needs to discuss and share their views, perceptions, and beliefs and come to an agreement of not only what happened but what are some of the ways of dealing with the difficulty they face. Otherwise, "*imposing* a reframe on clients they do not agree with can be disastrous" (p. 94). By this quote Figley is emphasizing the importance of having the family come to an agreement on what they must face and not trying to force one's beliefs upon the family.

Phase 4. Developing a healing theory. In this phase family members are called upon to consider all the elements of what happened to them, what they would do if faced with a similar situation in the future, what have been their interpretations and suggested solutions, and what, as a family, might be a constructive way of coping with and managing the current stressor or stressors they are encountering. Here the emphasis is on empowering the family on the direction for healing change and being careful again not to impose on them the therapist's views. The thoughtful, family-originated, strategy should arise and be scrutinized by all members of the family to reach a consensus on what can be done to get a hold of the problem or problems they face.

Phase 5. Involves closure and preparedness. During the final phase, the assistance of the therapist is terminated. The family recognizes that the goals of intervention have been reached and that they are the ones who have brought this about. The family has a sense of accomplishment and is in a far better position to deal with upcoming stressors and traumatic encounters that might arise. Families can be encouraged to be of assistance to other families who may be undergoing similar stressors. Thus, the family with an ill member or a family member traumatized by war experiences, natural disasters, assault, and many other forms of trauma can become a resource to other families, and in this way they may further embed the gains they have made.

Figley's strategies essentially involve empowerment of families so that they are in a stronger position to deal with the secondary traumatization they encounter. The strategy is not "therapy" per se but rather a facilitation or activation of families so that they are enabled to deal with the stultifying effects of secondary traumatization and to move forward toward an adaptive way of coping.

Another nontraditional approach to managing secondary trauma is presented by John Norcross.

## 7.3 Norcross Self-Care Strategies

Norcross (2000), in a summary of research findings on psychotherapist self-care, made several practical suggestions that could also be useful for those caring for ailing family members or performing their emotionally demanding obligations in their role as first responders or medical personnel. Among his suggestions, based on research findings, were the following:

1. Recognition of the hazards of the activity, whether it be therapy, medical treatment, police work, or other demanding social activity, is an important first step. "Affirming the universality of the hazards are in and of themselves therapeutic" (p. 710).
2. Employ strategies for ameliorating whatever the unique stressors might be. Possible strategies might be massage, meditation, yoga, exercise, peer support groups, and so on.
3. Self-awareness entails becoming aware of one's stressors and how one might traditionally cope with distress. Becoming self-aware might involve self-reflection or obtaining feedback from peers or significant others.
4. Employ multiple strategies and self-change skills as contrasted to sticking with one kind of approach.
5. Employ stimulus control and counterconditioning. Stimulus control might involve changing one's environment or setting so that it is less distressing, e.g., changing one's workspace or trying to make other changes in one's physical environment. By counterconditioning, Norcross is referring to action-oriented activities that produce diversion and relaxation such as moviegoing, engagement in a team sport, various forms of aerobic and anaerobic exercise, fishing, knitting, and any other activity that is uniquely relaxing and distracting to the individual who is secondarily traumatized.
6. Emphasize the human element. Here Norcross is suggesting that human contact and helping others can be stress-reducing, for example, peer groups, loving relationships and friendships, and participation in supervision groups.
7. Seeking therapy. This point is aimed specifically at psychotherapists but could also be of value to anyone else who finds themselves in emotionally depleting activities. Therapy need not be oriented to managing emotional disturbance as might be the goal of CBT but could simply involve the sharing of one's emotional concerns. The human contact and emotional unburdening can be of value for those who wish to do so.
8. Avoid wishful thinking and self-blame. Rather than hope that your job demands improve, it is suggested that taking any kind of action to bring change about is desirable. It is important not to be passive. Also, it is important that one not engage in self-criticism or self-blame for not being better able to manage overwhelming work demands.
9. Diversify. For therapists this might involve taking on varied kinds of cases and not only those focusing on traumatic experiences. For EMTs diversification might be taking time to train others or trying to change one's physical area of

responsibility. For physicians it might mean working with interns or becoming active in other medical specialties. For those caring for an ill family member, it might mean trying different strategies and approaches such as getting the ill person involved in video presentations or games, or reading to them, or seeking input from others, or obtaining more breaks in fulfilling one's responsibilities.
10. Appreciate the rewards. What is being suggested here is that secondary traumatization is often the outcome of giving of oneself in service of an important goal whether that goal is helping the community or assisting an ailing family member or keeping a segment of society safe and out of harm's way. It is suggested here that one focus one's attention on the importance and meaningfulness of these efforts. They are efforts aimed at helping others, and they are inherently worthy and worthwhile activities. In many ways the person engaging in the exhausting work of helping others is participating in noble work.

## 7.4 Gilbert-Eliot Strategies

Gilbert-Eliot (2020, p. 37), like Norcross (2000), has her own selection of what the title of her book refers to as "proven strategies" for managing the emotionally depleting consequences of secondary trauma. These strategies include the following:

1. Create a boundary between work and home. The suggestion here is to limit bringing work home from the office or place of work.
2. Change of lightened caseload/workload. For example, take on fewer assignments or cases until feeling more refreshed.
3. Schedule time off. The specific suggestion here is to schedule vacations and activities for holidays.
4. Meet or establish a peer group. The support and sharing with others are often beneficial in ameliorating the negative impact of secondary trauma. Here it is suggested that one join an existing peer group or form one if none exists.
5. Debrief with team or supervisor. Rather than continue the "daily grind," the author suggests meeting with the supervisor to go over and manage one's workload.
6. Change work schedule. An example here would be to try to schedule more difficult activities in the mornings when one has more energy. Obviously, one doesn't always have control over when demanding work obligations are scheduled.

## 7.5 Molnar et al. Strategies

Molnar et al. (2017), like the present author, conceptually combines compassion fatigue, secondary traumatic stress, and vicarious trauma (CF/STS/VT) as all essentially involving the costs of caring and suggests that self-directed, supportive, and other nontherapeutic approaches can be beneficial in both reducing the probability of developing secondary trauma but also of dealing with it once it occurs. Nevertheless, these authors cited Bober and Regehr (2006) who found that despite the widespread belief that engaging in self-care practices was helpful in managing secondary trauma, this did not necessarily translate into engaging in these practices, and when they were utilized, there was little indication of a reduction on trauma scores on standardized measures. Several of the reported interventions that were nevertheless reported as helpful in managing secondary trauma (Molnar et al., 2017) are the following:

1. Mindfulness-based stress reduction (MBSR) (Kabat-Zinn, 2003). This intervention is increasingly recommended as a way of decreasing secondary traumatic stress (e.g., Thieleman & Cacciatore, 2014) but is also of value in managing chronic pain, anxiety, depression, and daily stress. MBSR was initially used as a way of coping with chronic pain arising from serious illness. The essence of mindfulness is "paying attention in a particular way: on purpose, in the present moment, and non-judgmentally" (Kabat-Zinn, 1994, p. 4). Mindfulness trains one in focused attention so that one's mind does not wander to troubling thoughts that typically preoccupy an individual. In the case of secondary trauma, these thoughts would involve a focus on those traumatic experiences that others were enduring and one's own activities, thoughts, and preoccupations to ameliorate the distress. By engaging in mindfulness practices, one blocks or lessens the obsessive and consuming thoughts of trauma and its consequences and in that way lessens the impact of secondary trauma.
2. Affective and cognitive regulation. Miller and Sprang (2017) present a model for enhancing clinician experiences and reducing trauma. Here, emphasis is placed on affect and cognitive regulation and attention to parasympathetic functioning. There is a similarity between this approach and MBSR (Kabat-Zinn, 2003) in that one learns to focus attention on the present and to decrease mind-wandering and an obsessive focus on negative and traumatic experiences. Learning methods of controlling thoughts and reducing emotional distress thereby block the stunting impact of secondary trauma.
3. Professional skills training. It has been found that specific forms of training oriented toward dealing with traumatic stress-inducing situations and the subsequent perception that one has acquired these skills are associated with lower levels of secondary traumatization (Prati et al., 2010). Thus, perceptions of self-efficacy (Bandura, 1997) moderate the relationship between one's perceptions of stress and one's quality of life.
4. Psychoeducation. Berger and Gelkopf (2011) conducted a randomized controlled trial in which 90 pediatric nurses who worked in areas where war and terror were prevalent engaged in a 12-week program designed to identify trauma in infants and in young children. Families, including children when appropriate, were taught stress management techniques, as were the nurses, to better identify when stress was becoming unmanageable. The intervention was found to reduce secondary traumatic stress and improve perceptions of self-efficacy in compari-

son to waitlist controls. Similarly, Gentry et al. (2004) emphasized "training as treatment" as a way of improving one's competency in understanding and managing one's own secondary traumatic stress. The model stressed self-validation, connection, self-care, and other methods and found that there were decreases in secondary traumatic stress among a sample of 73 ER nurses.

5. Critical incident stress management (CISM) (Mitchell & Everly, 2000) and critical incident stress debriefing (CISD) (Mitchell, 1983) are based on the view that it is beneficial for those in stress responder roles to discuss or "debrief" feelings, perceptions, observations, and thoughts about traumatic encounters shortly after these occur. Such discussion is expected to ward off and prevent the development of negative embedded perceptions and beliefs about the traumatic encounters by processing them, typically in groups. These programs were first used in 1981 following a police shooting in Los Angeles and are based on the premise that peers and paraprofessionals trained within organizations are uniquely positioned to provide emotional support and to thereby avert subsequent drug and alcohol abuse as methods of coping with stress. There are few empirical studies to support these claims, but Stephens and Long (2000) did find an association between perceptions of social support and reductions in work-related traumatic stress in police officers. However, in the aftermath of a disaster or mass casualty, no evidence was found for the value of stress debriefing despite the opinion of its efficacy by experts (Fox et al., 2012). A similarly critical view is presented by Figley and Figley (2009) who report that the goal of CISD is to return the first responder to active duty, "rather than address the deeper issues of … the continuing traumatic reactions" (p. 177). Phipps and Byrne (2003) report that meta-analytic reviews find more support for CISM than CISD because the former incorporates the non-exposure-based strategies of CISD including muscle relaxation training, breathing retraining, alteration of internal dialogues, and thought stopping, all of which are components of stress inoculation training (SIT) (Michenbaum, 1985).

## 7.6 Phipps and Byrne Strategy

Phipps and Byrne (2003) recommend strategies that can be used by volunteer counseling organizations that might be of use to emergency service personnel, medical personnel, and those involved in other community-based services. It is important to note that these strategies are not psychotherapy per se but rather are approaches to be used in informal types of counseling. This "orienting approach" (p. 143) involves the following:

1. Supportive listening without eliciting details of the traumatic situation.
2. Using and accepting the secondarily or primarily traumatized individual's language for describing the traumatic situation.
3. Normalizing. Conveying to the trauma victim that their response was normal under the circumstances.

4. Teaching anxiety-reducing skills such as stress inoculation training (SIT) (Meichenbaum, 1985).
5. Providing practical advice such as where to find written information, self-help strategies, and professional therapeutic referral options if this is needed.

## 7.7 Summary

The use of structural interventions places an emphasis on practical approaches to managing secondary trauma that can be readily implemented. These approaches can lessen the negative impact of secondary traumatization without the need for individual psychotherapeutic interventions that might be used in cases involving PTSD. An array of strategies is presented, but there appear to be common elements among them. Some of these elements involve diversification of the care provider's intervention tasks, seeking activities that might take one away from one's preoccupations with the trauma of others, mindfulness practices, family counseling, trying to focus on the beneficial and enhancing outcomes of providing help to others, peer and social support groups, and so on. These strategies convey the view that secondary trauma is not a disorder per se but rather is akin to a common stress response arising from emotionally demanding activity. These emotionally demanding activities require specific strategies for their alleviation. The felt distress from engaging in these activities is not a "disorder" necessitating inclusion in a manual of psychiatric disorders (*DSM-5*, 2013). The following chapters will focus on additional strategies or activities that might be of value in the alleviation of the symptoms of secondary trauma.

# Chapter 8
# Social Support and Secondary Trauma

Like many other animals, humans are social beings. It might be said that we function best when we congregate, socialize, and function in various contexts within a pack or herd. According to Bryant (2021), "There is overwhelming evidence that social support is a hugely beneficial factor in reducing and coping with stress reactions" (p. 44). One might speculate that our evolutionary heritage selected out the need for social contact because social groups have a greater chance of survival than individuals in isolation. After many generations the need for social contact became genetically "hardwired" into us. When we oppose the biological imperative for social contact, such as when an individual is placed in solitary confinement, negative consequences abound. Research shows that the emotional distress of social isolation as a punishment can be as distressing as physical torture (e.g., Bosoglu et al., 2007; Reyes, 2007). The corollary also appears to be valid, that is, that social support has a distress-buffering or emotionally ameliorative effect (e.g., Bryant, 2021; Cohen & Wills, 1985; Ditzen & Heinrichs, 2014).

Social support is a complex topic (e.g., Stephens & Long, 2000), and our purpose is to focus on its stress-buffering aspects. Nevertheless, two broad categories of social support are the social structure of an individual's life and the functions served by interpersonal relationships. Structure is relevant to the degree to which a person is a part of a social network or networks. Functions include perceived social support, that is, the individual's perception of the kinds of support that are believed to be available. Some of these perceived types of support might include emotional support or one's belief that they have received empathy, caring, and so on. Other perceptions of social support can include the belief that one is supported by belonging to a social network and therefore has the availability of social engagement from others (Kent de Grey et al., 2018). Pennebaker (1997) suggests the positive impact of social support may be due to the promotion of the cognitive assimilation of troubling experiences by way of communicating and processing them and this serves to reduce rumination and flashbacks. In general, higher perceived social support is frequently associated with positive mental health outcomes and with desirable physical health consequences such as lower rates of cardiovascular disease and lower mortality (House et al., 1988).

© The Author(s), under exclusive license to Springer Nature Switzerland AG 2023

R. W. Motta, *Secondary Trauma*, https://doi.org/10.1007/978-3-031-44308-4_8

## 8.1 Rob Seeks a Social Support Group

In Chap. 4, we encountered the case of Rob and Laura. Rob had met and fallen in love with Laura, married, and they decided to have a child. After having met with a fertility specialist to find out why Laura was not becoming pregnant, it was discovered that she had what ultimately turned out to be a cancerous tumor of the breast. After years of a variety of different types of cancer treatments, some of which involved agonizing high-dose chemotherapy, Laura passed away. Rob was traumatized by witnessing Laura's emotional and physical pain and that of her family, and he was devastated by her loss. On the day of her death, as Rob was leaving the hospital in a state of bewildered despair, a compassionate nurse told him of a support group and handed him a pamphlet. Rob thought the chances of him joining or deriving any comfort from such a group was nonexistent. Two weeks later, still in a state of tormented gloom, Rob picked up the pamphlet, called the enclosed number, and scheduled attendance at a meeting.

The group was run by a social worker, and the meeting appeared to be a combined secondary trauma, primary trauma, and bereavement group. There was an abundance of emotional and physical pain in this group and an assortment of diagnoses, but all of these were connected to some form of cancer. Most of the groups were family members of someone who was currently suffering from or recently died of some form of cancer. Many of the cancers that Rob heard about in the group were alien to him, such as leiomyosarcoma, non-Hodgkin's lymphoma, cholangiocarcinoma, Kaposi sarcoma, mesothelioma, and others. Rob's first impression was, "Who the hell needs this? The last thing I need is to hear about other people's sorrows." He was convinced that he had made a mistake, and although he informed the group leader that he would return, he did not think he would. It was all too much to bear.

By the time Rob returned home, he realized that there was something vaguely comforting about the cancer group he had attended. It made him feel less isolated and less disconnected from the world. The social worker who led the group appeared to do little more than encourage people to reveal what had happened to them and to report any new developments that were now taking place. She did not seem to be employing any specific therapeutic technique other than the facilitation of communication. The following week Rob returned to the group and agreed to reveal the details about his situation involving his and Laura's desire to have a child then being confronted with the existence of a cancer that appeared to be, and was, unstoppable. His and Laura's decade-long fight against cancer elicited a good deal of sympathetic head nodding and sincere expressions of empathy from the members of the group.

Rob attended this group weekly for the full 2 months that it had been scheduled to run. Years later he continued to report that he found the group helpful in dealing with the emotional pain and loss he had endured. He claims that he still has vivid images of Laura's suffering. One image that keeps coming back to him is Laura lying in a hospital bed with 12 intravenous lines running into her body. Some were for hydration, some for chemotherapy, some for nausea, and some to fight infection, and there were others whose functions were unknowable to him. He recalls Laura's weakness and fatigue brought on by the cancer and by narcotics to deaden her pain. Despite the continuing clarity of these painful images, Rob reports that the group somehow made the memories less painful for him. It is unclear to him exactly what within the group he found so helpful. He finally concluded that the group made him feel that his pain was understood by others and that he was not alone. There was something unidentifiably beneficial in the social support that the group provided. The social support of the group itself, independent of what the group leader did, appeared to Rob to be the primary ingredient that helped him. The concept that we are "wired" to be social beings is likely why Rob found this support group to be so helpful. Human beings are social animals who function well in "packs." Social support is a uniquely therapeutic factor in alleviating experienced distress (Williams, 1993).

## 8.2 Help for Helpers

Emergency medical services personnel such as emergency medical dispatchers are often confronted with significant levels of stress in their contacts with those who are undergoing traumatic experiences. They take calls requiring the need for ambulance services, paramedics, emergency medical technicians, and so on. These calls are often desperate cries for assistance and dispatchers must provide telephonic support until assistance arrives on the scene. Frequently, they provide medical advice, psychological support, and nonprofessional supportive counseling, all of which they are minimally trained to give. They often develop secondary traumatization because of their job demands and from inherent organizational and operational pressures (Brough, 2005; Kirby et al., 2011).

Shakespeare-Finch et al. (2015) conducted a study that evaluated 60 individuals involved in emergency dispatch work. Participants completed measures of social support, self-efficacy, or the degree that they felt effective and competent at their job (Bandura, 1997), psychological well-being, and a trauma-related measure that assesses the degree to that one's thoughts are intruded upon by traumatic memories, that is, the Impact of Events Scale-Revised (IES-R; Weiss & Marmar, 1997). Among the findings were that social support and perceptions of self-efficacy were found to be significant predictors of well-being. Receiving social support was also found to reduce trauma-related reactions and to also contribute to posttraumatic growth (Tedeschi & Calhoun, 1996). Receiving lower levels of social support was associated with higher levels of trauma reactions.

The authors note limitations of the study such as its cross-sectional nature and reliance on self-report measures. They also note that respondents are prone to the memory biases that induce them to present answers in a socially desirable manner (Bauhoff, 2011). Nevertheless, this type of research is difficult to conduct without relying on self-report. The validity of the study's findings is comparable to other studies showing that social support reduces the negative psychological impact of trauma. Shakespeare-Finch's outcome data are in accord with Williams (1993) who states, "The single most effective method for resolution of traumatic stress is talking about the trauma with others who went through it … Our experience has been that the support of coworkers during the weeks following the trauma is vital to resolution" (p. 932).

## 8.3 Social Support Among First Responders

First responders such as police officers, firefighters, paramedics, and others often encounter secondary traumatization owing to their attempts at resolving traumatic situations in the civilian world. It was indicated in Chap. 5 that while this work is frequently associated with secondary trauma, many of these groups also experience posttraumatic growth and are esteemed by the communities they serve. This positive feedback is also received by police officers, but they can carry the burden of social disapproval owing to press disclosures of brutality and discrimination against groups representing diversity. These additional pressures on police officers were previously stated to have resulted in an increased level of early retirements and resignations. A comprehensive study of the value of social support in ameliorating traumatic stress in police officers was conducted by Stephens and Long (2000).

The Stephens and Long study specifically examined the stress-buffering effects of communication with police supervisors and peers. The study involved 527 police officers from various ranks and investigated both content and ease of communication. The study examined the impact of social support on psychological symptoms, such as jumpiness and preoccupation with stressful events; physical symptoms, such as body aches, dizziness, and headaches; and traumatic events, such as experiencing robbery, physical assault, sexual assault, motor vehicle crash, natural disaster, and fire.

Among the findings of the Stephens and Long study was that a significant association was found among the experience of work-related stressors and psychological and physical difficulties. It was also found that higher levels of social support, as measured by the amount of communication, buffered the relationship between stressors and psychological or physical health outcomes, but these findings were only relevant to certain forms of communication. Perceptions of ease of communication with peers about traumatic experiences at work, communications about disturbing experiences, and positive and negative communications about work and peers were found to have the most stress-buffering effects. However, too much communication was found to have a "reverse buffering effect" (p. 419). In other words, moderate levels of communication with peers were helpful, but intense levels were not. In contrast to communication with peers, "most of the supervisor communication variables did not buffer the trauma-strain relationship" (p. 421), although some degree of stress buffering was found when communication with supervisors involved complaints about work and work conditions. Overall findings of the study showed that one's perceptions of ease of communication with peers, engaged in at a moderate level, had the most beneficial effects on perceived stress and psychological or physical symptoms related to police work. This study showed that social support can be beneficial in ameliorating secondary traumatic stress among police officers and that there are moderating factors including ease and intensity of communication and whether the communication is with peers or supervisors. Ease and availability of communication with peers, but not typically with supervisors, were the most beneficial forms of social support. Similar findings have been reported by other researchers who show that "interpersonal resources" (e.g., Salston & Figley, 2003) mitigate the impact of secondary traumatization arising from a variety of causes.

## 8.4 Social Support Barriers

The Stephens and Long (2000) study and other such studies of the beneficial impact of peer support among first responders provide us with information on the types of support that are helpful in ameliorating secondary traumatic stress. One of the major problems that police officers, and perhaps other uniformed services, face is that seeking help runs counter to the self and social image of those in first responder roles. Military personnel, police officers, firefighters, and others are part of a culture that often views help-seeking as a sign of weakness (Motta, 2020, 2021). There is a subculture of police officers that involves its own rules, behavioral expectations, language, and mentality (Woody, 2005, 2006). Rudofossi (2007), for example, states, "At the police academy, open expression of fear was unacceptable, and skepticism of any sort was considered resistance" (p. 24). This mentality continues after the candidate graduates from the academy, and it becomes part of the identity of many first responders. Even though the police and other uniformed services have a sense of security arising out of feelings of being enculturated into a brotherhood of strong, independent people upon whom others rely for their safety, the emotional expression of fear or reports of being traumatized are simply unacceptable. Not only is there an intolerance of the perceived "weakness" in those who seek help, but there is also an intolerance of one's own fears and needs for assistance. While there may be employee assistance programs for many of the uniformed services, seeking this help is simply not part of their culture. Seeking help runs so counter to the first responder culture in that it is seen as weakness, and it might even result in the blocking of promotion (Motta, 2020).

Another barrier to seeking help and social support for those who have experienced secondary trauma or PTSD, and particularly those of the uniformed services, is avoidance of memories of the trauma. "Avoidance is the most common way in which people deal with distressing situations" (Motta, 2020, pp. 11–12). Most forms of treatment for psychological trauma involve some form of review and reprocessing of traumatic events. The more realistic this reengaging in traumatic memories is, the more effective the treatment (e.g., Foa et al., 2007; Foa & Kozak, 1986), but unfortunately this realism often elicits so much anxiety that social support and other forms of treatment are avoided along with those therapists or peer counselors who provide this support. Peer counselors and others who attempt to provide support are well-meaning but often lack the knowledge that moving too quickly in helping the person who is seeking assistance can activate an avoidance response and the secondary trauma victim then will flee treatment. It is important to heed the warning of trauma theorist Peter Levine who advises that one can never move too slowly in treating trauma (Levine, 2010) so as not to activate this anxiety-avoidance response.

## 8.5 Professional Care Providers: The Case of Dr. Thiel

When Dr. Thiel, a psychiatrist, arrived for counseling, it was evident that she was on a mission to treat those who were experiencing PTSD due to war experiences. She worked primarily for the Veterans Administration Health Services and occasionally taught a course in abnormal psychology at a local community college. Most of her caseloads were aged veterans of the Vietnam War, a war where she had served as a medic decades ago. She did not have much actual combat experience but rather worked in field hospitals that were distant from combat engagements. After completion of her tour of duty, she enrolled in medical school and ultimately specialized in psychiatry. She indicated that despite her medical training, she was aware that the antidepressants and the antianxiety agents that are typically prescribed for PTSD were of little value but that she had found counseling to be far more effective. Dr. Thiel stated that the reason she was seeking help was that she was finding herself increasingly depressed, irritable, and preoccupied with the PTSD cases she was treating.

Dr. Thiel's therapist, Dr. Silva, is a licensed psychologist who, like Dr. Thiel, attended professional school after having served his time in an army helicopter unit based in Bien Hoa, South Vietnam. Dr. Thiel had sought out this therapist because of his war experience and because he regularly treated civilian cases of PTSD. She was not seeking traditional therapy for PTSD per se but rather was seeking emotional support from someone who had a background like hers. Dr. Silva informed Dr. Thiel that for their talks to be helpful, they would have to involve at least some reviewing and reprocessing of the cases Dr. Thiel had treated, especially those involving traumatic experiences related to war. Dr. Silva assured Dr. Thiel that he would move slowly to not overwhelm her with anxiety.

During the next session, Dr. Thiel began relating a case that she had found particularly agonizing. As she began detailing her sessions with a particular veteran who was in his 70s, she appeared to become increasingly upset. Dr. Silva, being aware of Levine's (2010) dictum of the need to move slowly when treating trauma, attempted to divert Dr. Thiel and have her discuss more neutral and less anxiety-provoking material. But Dr. Thiel could not hold herself back. She immediately immersed herself in a discussion of the treatment of a veteran who shot and killed what he thought was an "enemy soldier" while the veteran was "walking point."

Walking point involves walking ahead of a group of soldiers to alert and thereby protect the group from being ambushed. Walking point is an extremely anxiety-provoking although necessary activity whereby one soldier puts him or herself in harm's way for the protection of a larger group.

Dr. Thiel related that this soldier was walking slowly through the jungle with a heightened sense of alertness when he spotted what appeared to be movement in the surrounding vegetation. Certain that this had to be an enemy soldier prowling through the jungle, he brought his M-16 rifle to eye level and fired a burst of rounds. He heard a yell and then silence. As he and members of the group he was leading came upon the scene of the shooting, they were horrified to see that the "enemy soldier" that had been shot and killed was a pregnant woman from one of the local villages. They were all stunned but were also aware that the anxiety of walking point sometimes led to panicked weapons firing. Civilian casualties are a dreaded consequence of all wars, and this war was no exception. There was no investigation that followed on from this accidental killing of an unarmed and pregnant civilian especially because the nearby village from which she came had been suspected of harboring enemy soldiers. After leaving the army, the soldier was tortured by this event, and his torment went on for decades until he began seeing Dr. Thiel at the Veterans Health Services Administration.

Dr. Thiel was now sobbing as she related her own secondary traumatization that resulted from treating this tormented client. She related that she was often plagued by nightmares and sleeplessness particularly on those days when she had therapy sessions with this veteran. Dr. Silva assured her that her symptoms were commonly seen in therapists who deal with trauma and that the continued reprocessing of her secondary trauma experiences would likely lead to the alleviation of her distress.

At their next appointment, Dr. Silva waited patiently as the minutes ticked away and Dr. Thiel did not appear in the waiting area. The following day he called Dr. Thiel and she informed him that the distress she experienced in the session that they had together made her secondary trauma symptoms dramatically worse and that she would not come back for further sessions. Dr. Silva informed her that elevated distress is common when recounting secondary trauma memories, but none of this reasoning had any impact on Dr. Thiel and she did not return. She simply found the session with Dr. Silva so distressing that she could not continue with her social support sessions.

This case illustrates that while social and therapeutic support can be helpful in treating secondary trauma, it can also fail to help because of the unintended distress elevation that it can cause. There are other situations in which intended social support proves unhelpful. For example, there are instances in which the cultural ethos of helpers and providers interferes with seeking and obtaining help. Providers often believe that they should be strong and capable of helping others. Help-seeking for themselves is often not a part of this ethos. At other times, as in the case of Dr. Thiel, the anxiety and distress that arise from confronting secondary trauma is a major barrier to treatment success. In addition, avoidance of social support in general is a common response among those who acquire primary and secondary trauma, despite the value of social support and therapy. "Participants who enter therapy with strong tendencies of avoid aversive events, not surprisingly, tend to avoid the demands of therapy by dropping out …" (Bryant et al., 2007, p. 15). Thus, while social support, whether provided by peers or professionals, can and often does, alleviate the symptoms of secondary trauma, there are instances in which help-seeking is avoided or is seen as unhelpful.

Two months after Dr. Thiel stopped seeing Dr. Silva, the latter received a call from Dr. Thiel. She informed Dr. Silva that she had joined a social support group of psychologists, social workers, and another psychiatrist. The group stayed away from the discussion of specific cases that were in treatment but rather focused on the impact of therapeutic work on the provider's daily functioning. Dr. Thiel indicated that she found this group helpful and far less overwhelming than the treatment she had received from Dr. Silva that involved discussion of cases. She stated that she appreciated Dr. Silva's efforts but wanted him to know that she simply could not handle delving into individual cases. It was apparent from this call that social support can be effective in managing secondary trauma, but the focus needed to be on general peer support and not immersion into specific traumatizing experiences. Dr. Silva was once again reminded of the fact that in treating trauma, it is important to move slowly.

## 8.6 Summary

This chapter begins with a discussion of interventions for secondary traumatization and takes the position that social support has been shown to have a distress-buffering effect and that our responsiveness to such support appears to be "hardwired" into us. The chapter also presents barriers or factors that can reduce the effectiveness of social support interventions. These barriers include the resistance to seeking out and receiving social support because seeking help may suggest weakness. Seeking help also goes against the ethos of many of the uniformed services who tend to see themselves as strong and self-reliant. In some cases, the seeking of support can potentially reduce the chances of advancement in one's chosen field. Case presentations are made involving social support for secondary trauma due to family illness, to the job demands of first responders, and to the burdens carried by professional caregivers. The chapter also takes a closer look at the nature of social support and concludes that moderate amounts of sharing of one's secondary traumatic stress can be beneficial whereas excessive sharing can have an "anti-stress-buffering" effect. Similarly, it is shown that the persons with whom trauma-relevant information is shared can affect the buffering character of social support. Sharing with peers was shown to be helpful, while sharing with supervisors did not result in beneficial effects. Overall, social support does appear to be an empirically validated way of managing the distress due to secondary traumatization. Future chapters will examine other empirically supported approaches to lessening the impact of secondary traumatization.

# Chapter 9
# Exercise and Secondary Trauma

There is substantial literature supporting the role of exercise in reducing distress of various kinds, including anxiety, depression, and stress-related disorders (e.g., Bernstein & McNally, 2017; Strohle, 2009). Regarding secondary trauma, regular aerobic activity appears to foster resilience and dampen excessive emotional reactivity due to stress, regardless of whether this stress is due to compassion fatigue or other factors (Flueckiger et al., 2016; Kishida & Elavsky, 2015). In general, those who exercise regularly have been found to be better able to cope with stressors than those who do not (Southwick et al., 2005). For that reason, exercise can be a valuable resource for those whose activities, whether familial or professional, eventuate in secondary traumatization. The question of why exercise, particularly aerobic exercise, is so helpful in managing stress, anxiety, depression, and other negative emotional states remains, for the most part, unanswered. Several theoretical positions have been put forward to explain positive exercise effects.

## 9.1 Physiological Hypotheses of Exercise Effects

***Thermogenic Hypothesis*** This hypothesis proposes that the known benefits of exercise are due to physical activity's elevation of body temperature (e.g., DeBoer et al., 2012). It is believed that temperature elevation, particularly in the brain stem, is associated with tranquilizing effects and especially with reductions in anxiety. There are several problems with this hypothesis including the possibility that temperature elevation may be a mediating or moderating variable and that the actual causal agent might be some other influences, for example, neurochemical changes. In this case temperature elevation would serve a correlational but not a causal role. Further if temperature elevation was the cause of anxiety reduction, one would expect to see a relationship between fever or warm climates and reduced anxiety, and this is not the case. The thermogenic hypothesis has not held up well as an explanatory construct of exercise benefits.

© The Author(s), under exclusive license to Springer Nature Switzerland AG 2023 
R. W. Motta, *Secondary Trauma*, https://doi.org/10.1007/978-3-031-44308-4_9

***Endorphin and Endocannabinoid Hypotheses*** The endorphin hypothesis (e.g., Farrell et al., 1982) is probably the most popular and widely accepted explanation as to why exercise has stress-reducing effects. This in no way implies that it is the correct explanation but simply that it initially captured the interest of researchers, but now it has been the target of multiple critiques. It had been found that when one engages in vigorous exercise, there is an accompanying elevation in the endogenous opiate, beta-endorphin. Later studies appeared to contradict this explanation, and like the thermogenic hypothesis, it has been suggested that beta-endorphin levels might be correlates rather than causes of the beneficial impact on stress and occurrence of the "runner's high" (e.g., Motta, 2018). For example, Alfermann and Stoll (2005) demonstrated that a jogging group, a relaxation group, and a stretching group all demonstrated reductions in negative states such as anger, stress, tension, and elevations in calmness and positive mood. If there is a link between exercise, beta-endorphin level, and positive affect, then the non-exercise groups should not have shown positive psychological effects.

Further critiques of the popular endorphin hypothesis exist. These include the fact that naloxone, an opiate antagonist, does not block the runner's high, and it should if endorphin elevation is the cause of improved mood states. Finally, circulating blood endorphins are not strongly related to brain level endorphins as endorphins do not cross the blood-brain barrier. Affective states are primarily seen as due to brain influences, but endorphin levels after exercise are not taken from the brain, and therefore body sampled blood levels of endorphins cannot account for mood elevation that is seen in vigorous exercise (Motta, 2020).

An alternative to the endorphin hypothesis is called the endocannabinoid hypothesis (Smaga et al., 2014). Endocannabinoids are lipid-based neurotransmitters normally produced by the body and, unlike endorphins, do appear to operate both centrally (i.e., in the brain) and peripherally. These substances are similar in action to tetrahydrocannabinol or THC, the active ingredient in marijuana, and produce analgesic effects that might be an explanation for the runner's high, that is, the reduction of perceived emotional distress following running, and other beneficial psychological effects such as anxiety reduction. To some extent, both the endorphin and endocannabinoid hypotheses are suggestive of an unlikely single-cause explanation for why exercise appears to result in positive psychological effects. It is possible that the endocannabinoid interpretation of positive exercise effects represents a more defensible alternative to the endorphin explanation because of the former's ability to operate in both the central and peripheral nervous systems. Further research is needed regarding the role of endocannabinoids in stress reduction, but it is possible and perhaps likely that they, like endorphins, might be correlated with exercise and that some other system or systems are what underlies the benefits of exercise.

***Monoamine Hypothesis*** The monoamine hypothesis is like the endorphin and endocannabinoid hypotheses in that it suggests that exercise is responsible for the production of certain neurotransmitters, in this case, serotonin, dopamine, and norepinephrine, and that their production is associated with psychologically beneficial effects such as reductions in depression (e.g., Lin & Kuo, 2013). These neurotransmitters are found to be elevated following exercise and are typically detected through evaluation of urine and blood plasma. The problem with this mode of evaluation is that urine and blood samples do not necessarily reflect the levels of these substances in the brain. A further problem is that to assess possible brain levels of neurotransmitters more accurately, invasive procedures such as spinal taps for the acquisition of cerebrospinal fluids are often necessary (e.g., Martinsen, 1987). The difficulty in doing this with large samples of participants as would be necessary in research studies presents obvious hurdles. As a result, consistent findings that would support the monoamine hypothesis are not available (Patki et al., 2014).

An additional problem that plagues each of the neurophysiological and neurochemical hypotheses and is a difficulty for most other efforts to assess the connection between exercise and psychological states is that the assessment of such states requires some form of self-report and, thus, subjectivity. These self-reports are vulnerable to sources of error that have been variously labeled as experimenter bias effects, expectancy effects, observer expectancy effects, social desirability responding, and others. For example, a participant in such a study might be required to exercise and then be questioned or asked to complete questionnaires or other paper-and-pencil measures that assess their emotional status. Because it is commonly known that exercise produces beneficial psychological effects, the participants might, consciously or unconsciously, provide the experimenter with what they believe the experimenter wants, which is a report of an elevated or positive mood state or decreases in negative affect such as anxiety and depression. The reliance on the self-report of exercise study participants introduces a kind of error that is difficult to control regardless of the nature of the study being conducted.

## 9.2 Psychological Hypotheses of Exercise Effects

***Distraction Hypothesis*** The essence of the distraction hypothesis of exercise is that exercise allows one to put at least a temporary halt to the ruminations typically seen in those who are depressed and/or who are experiencing stressors linked to various sources including secondary traumatization. In fact, the reduction of depressive rumination was found to be tied to exercise activities such as cycling (Bernstein & McNally, 2017) and to be a significant factor in arming one against future depression. In the Bernstein et al. study, exercise activity was shown to have a dampening effect on depressive rumination that occurred in response to subsequent stressors. In other words, exercise was found to not only lessen depression but to arm exercisers against future depression in response to stressors. A central contributing factor responsible for depression was found in the Bernstein et al. study to be rumination. Similar findings regarding the contributory role of depressive rumination to negative affect have been reported by Nolen-Hoeksema et al. (2008).

Distracting activities such as assertiveness training, relaxation, social contact, and others have also been investigated in studies where they are compared with exercise, but results have been inconclusive, with exercise being more effective than some of these activities and similar to other activities regarding the reduction in depressive affect (e.g., Martinsen et al., 1989). However, when one examines mood elevation and not simply the reduction in depressive affect, it does appear that exercise does have more impact than activities such as relaxation or waitlist controls (Alfermann & Stoll, 2005). An overall examination of the specific factors inherent in exercise activity that result in beneficial psychological effects continues to elude investigators. According to Craft and Perna (2004), the underlying mechanisms of the depression-reducing effects of exercise remain unclear. Distraction is likely to be a partial contributor to exercise benefits and can be of value for those whose compassion fatigue and secondary traumatization leave them preoccupied and ruminating, and, in that way, it is a valuable tool for providing emotional escape and relief.

***Self-Efficacy Hypothesis*** Another explanation for the stress-reducing characteristics of exercise is the self-efficacy hypothesis, named by its popularizer, Albert Bandura (1997). Bandura claimed that people who are depressed, as is often the case in situations involving secondary traumatization, appear to have lowered self-perceptions of their capability to achieve their objectives. These people appear to feel comparatively powerless in comparison to their non-distressed, nondepressed peers. Self-efficacy refers to one's perceptions of their capability to achieve objectives, and available research shows that exercise is an effective activity for lowering depression and presumably enhancing self-efficacy perceptions (e.g., Bernstein & McNally, 2017).

A control group study involving 19 adults suffering from formerly diagnosed clinical depression and who participated in an exercise program was carried out by Craft (2005). This quasi-experimental design study involved 9 weeks of moderately intense exercise sessions lasting 20 min and conducted three to four times per week. The exercise included activities such as brisk walking or using a stationary cycle ergometer or treadmill. A series of measures were completed after the third and ninth week of exercise. The findings of the study were that those in the exercise group showed significant reductions in depression at the 9-week assessment period in comparison to controls. The exercise group participants also showed enhancement of self-efficacy perceptions and reductions in depressive rumination like that which was seen in the Bernstein et al. study (2017) reported above. Also seen at the 9-week assessment were increases in perceived coping self-efficacy. The latter finding suggests that moderate exercise produced enhanced perceptions of the ability to cope in general. One can see the value of this in relation to secondary traumatization. Those who experience secondary traumatic stress often feel overwhelmed and experience a decreased ability to cope with the demands that are being placed on them. If exercise enhances self-perceptions of general coping ability, this can be of significant benefit for those who feel emotionally drained and exhausted from supportive roles they play, whether this involves family demands or the giving of first responders or health-care providers. Like the Bernstein et al. study (2017), Craft (2005) emphasized the important role played by the reduction in depressive rumination in reducing depressive affect. In summary this study provided evidence for exercise having multiple effects including enhancement of perceived coping ability, reduction in depression, and reduction in depressive rumination.

***Bodymind Hypothesis as a Synthesis*** It could be argued that the mind-body separation or "dualism" of Descartes (1596–1650) is countered by the twentieth-century bodymind hypothesis of Candace Pert. This hypothesis may be seen as a synthesis of the physiological and psychological hypotheses for explaining why exercise may have beneficial effects. The term *bodymind* was coined by Candace Pert, a psychopharmacologist and neuroscientist. Pert is well-known for having described natural or endogenous opioids within the body. These endogenous opioids are a group of neuropeptides or small chains of amino acids that are synthesized and released by neurons (Pert et al., 1985) and that are said to underlie, or be associated with, many psychological states, including positive effects that follow from exercise.

The bodymind hypothesis differs from the concept of mind-body interaction in that the latter implies a causality whereby body states affect emotional states and emotional states can impact the body. An example of a mind-body relationship can be seen when the unremitting stress of secondary traumatization causes a weakening of the immune system. An emotional state of distress dampens the physiological state of immune function. A primary difference between mind-body interaction and bodymind is that the latter suggests that there are no separate states of mind and body but rather there is a single entity and that it does not make neurophysiological sense to speak of the states separately. In the case example above the bodymind hypothesis would view secondary trauma and immune system response as occurring simultaneously. One's neurochemistry and one's psychological status are therefore inextricably united. As a result, a bodymind formulation would not be used to explain *why* exercise results in psychological benefits. Instead, one might say, as did the Roman poet Juvenal (60–130 CE), mens sana in corpore sano—a healthy mind in a healthy body; that is, mind states and body states are inseparable. In the bodymind interpretation of exercise and its positive psychological effects, we see that there is no causality. There is a unity by which benefits from exercise are reflected in both body and mind, or bodymind. There are no body states or mind states only bodymind states. Pert's concept of bodymind essentially eliminates the need for seeking causal mechanisms for the beneficial effects of exercise.

***Conclusions Regarding Hypotheses of Exercise Effects*** Each of the hypothesized mechanisms that theoretically underlie the value of exercise as a way of coping with negative affect, such as that seen in secondary traumatization, appears to have some level of empirical support, although the thermogenic hypothesis seems the least supported. None of the hypotheses offers incontestable conclusions, and none are invulnerable to the possibility that alternative interpretations of why exercise is associated with stress and depression reduction. The bodymind hypothesis makes the seeking of cause unnecessary. Despite the bodymind view, it is possible that some yet-to-be-identified factor or factors account for the benefits of exercise and the physiologically and psychologically based hypotheses are simply correlated with those factors. It is also possible that all the hypotheses come into play on some level such that there are multiple mechanisms involved in considering the beneficial effects of exercise. Another interpretation of exercise effects is that the various hypotheses are each valid depending on where in one's cycle of emotional distress one chooses to conduct an assessment (Motta, 2020). At this point, there appears to be no definitive and universally accepted answer to the question of why exercise has a positive psychological impact on those who are experiencing distress and depression. What we do know is that the available research does support the value of exercise, whether aerobic or non-aerobic in reducing emotional distress, and for this reason, exercise can be of value in alleviating the strains of secondary traumatization.

## 9.3 Mishal and Secondary Trauma

Mishal was born into a well-to-do Muslim family in Iran, and overall, she was a happy child who had many friends and did well in school. She was from a close and loving family, and as was their cultural tradition, at age 15, a marriage was arranged for her with a man, Afsar, 20 years her senior. His name can be translated as "commander," which in Afsar's case was appropriate because at the time he was a captain in the Iranian army. The marriage was stable, but Mishal had some difficulty getting close to Afsar as he tended toward being autocratic and he rarely complimented her. As Afsar rose in the military ranks and eventually attained the rank of general, Mishal took care of the three boys that they eventually had together. Afsar's ascent in the ranks was not without difficulty as his somewhat politically liberal views clashed with those of his far more conservative superiors. Knowing that his career had stalled and that he might be accused of disloyalty or even subversiveness, a decision was made to move to the USA. Another reason for moving was that their youngest son, who was then 13, had been diagnosed as having Type A diabetes and there was a hope that he might be better treated in the USA than in Iran.

Once in the USA, Afsar found work as a consultant at a security agency that provided services to banks. Mishal, needing an escape from her increasingly autocratic husband, the demands of motherhood, and especially the worries about her youngest son's health, enrolled in classes to become an assistant physical therapist. Although absorbed by classwork, practicum, and internship assignments, Mishal had difficulty escaping the burdens of her somewhat distant marriage, but she was especially burdened by what she viewed as her younger son, Farid's, difficulties adjusting to his illness. Farid often complained bitterly about having to check his insulin levels four times a day, to inject insulin, to watch what he ate, making sure that he did not consume too many carbohydrates and that he adhered to a plant-based diet. But most of all Farid deplored and complained bitterly about not being like everyone else who did not have this autoimmune disease that was attacking his pancreas. Mishal became increasingly preoccupied and distressed by Farid and his difficulties. She suffered from nightmares and did not see her husband as providing much in the way of emotional support. As an immigrant in the USA, she did not feel that there was much social support for her even among the friends that she did have. The combination of an unsupportive marriage, living in a strange land, and most of all dealing with a child who was both troubled by his illness and often resistant to keeping a watchful eye on his blood sugar status burdened Mishal to such a degree that she sought counseling for what was said to be secondary trauma. Her husband, Afsar, did not approve of counseling and criticized Mishal for what he saw as weakness. He believed that people should be able to manage their own problems and not rely on counseling, which he viewed with suspicion and as an American form of self-absorption.

Mishal felt that the psychologist she was seeing helped her to develop a greater sense of self-worth and supported her in her vocational goals. Nevertheless, Mishal continued to feel unhappily burdened by what she saw as the suffering of her younger son, her remote and critical husband, and the difficulties adjusting to a country that would always be a foreign land to her. Her developing depression led her to a psychiatric consultation and this to a trial on the antidepressant Lexapro. Along the way Mishal also tried yoga, meditation, and daily brisk walks. These combined interventions did result in an improvement in Mishal's mood state, and she developed a sense of fulfillment in having obtained a position at a local physical therapy clinic where she was seen as a valued staff member.

Farid eventually had gone off to college and was finishing the fall semester of his sophomore year. He continued to have a great deal of difficulty accepting that he had a lifelong diabetic condition that required constant monitoring and moderating of insulin levels. This difficulty translated into his frequently ignoring his condition despite medical advice and using alternative approaches such as regular exercise, stress reduction and relaxation exercises, and eating a diet virtually devoid of processed foods and having severe restrictions on carbohydrates. In the latter part of December of his second year, following the completion of his final exams, Farid went to his dorm room in a disoriented state. He was found dead the next morning having previously lapsed into a diabetic coma.

Mishal, Afsar, and their two other and now adult children were devastated by their loss of Farid. Regrettably, Afsar dealt with this tragedy by becoming even more remote and withdrawn, but his desperation over the loss of his son was obvious. He seldom spoke to Mishal about the death of Farid, and Mishal interpreted his silence as a tacit form of blame because she believed that Afsar viewed the care of children as a mother's "duty." Late December is now typically an unhappy time for Mishal and triggers an intense anniversary reaction of depression.

In a case like this where Mishal was receiving psychotherapy, psychotropic medication, and participating in yoga, meditation, and exercise, it is difficult to determine which of these interventions was most helpful. It is likely that for everyone who deals with a unique set of stressors, different interventions might be seen as more helpful than others, and maybe the choice of the most effective intervention might vary over time. When Mishal was asked, her response was that the one activity that she would not give up was her brisk walking. She stated that no matter how troubled she felt at the start of her walk, she always returned to a better mental state.

Mishal's walking usually began at 6:30 in the morning and took place every day. She walked for about an hour and covered approximately 3 miles and sometimes more. Mishal stated that walking was much like prayer. It was something she did faithfully and regularly. She valued the solitude on her walks. She did not seek social support or social contact when exercising. Sometimes she listened to music through her earbuds, but most of the time, it was walking alone in the peaceful quiet of the early morning that gave her the strength to not only get through her days but to do so with some degree of equanimity and contentment. To this day her relationship with her husband continues to be remote, and in fact they sleep in separate bedrooms. They do share one meal together in the evenings but mostly they lead separate lives. Mishal has come to accept her marriage as it is, enjoys her physical therapy work, and feels that she has a wonderful and fulfilling relationship with her two "boys." Regular exercise through brisk early morning walking is Mishal's "best medicine." She claims that she plans to continue her energetic walks until she is unable to do so. Brisk walking is the elixir that has allowed Mishal to manage a series of difficulties that just about anyone would find daunting. It is reasonable to say the exercise has become the medicine that keeps Mishal going and that keeps her fulfilled. Why exercise would be so beneficial for her in comparison to her other activities of counseling, medication, yoga, and meditation is an unanswerable question. What is clear, however, is that for Mishal the aerobic exercise of brisk walking has, according to her, provided substantial aid in prevailing over her difficulties.

## 9.4 Studies of Exercise as a Trauma Intervention

While it may be of interest to speculate as to the hypothetical underpinnings of why exercise has beneficial psychological effects, these are more the concerns of academics than of clinicians. The clinician, although recognizing the value of exercise in managing depression, anxiety, and stress due to secondary traumatization, is often hard-pressed to get a distressed client to engage in exercise at all. Mulcahy (1988), for example, conducted a study in which individuals diagnosed with major depressive disorder were assigned to one of two groups. In group one, participants engaged in CBT for 6 weeks, followed by 6 weeks of aerobic exercise, which was primarily brisk walking and jogging. Group two did the reverse. They engaged in 6 weeks of exercise followed by 6 weeks of CBT. The main findings of the study were twofold. First, both CBT alone and exercise alone resulted in statistically significant reductions in the levels of depression. Post-intervention depression levels were reduced below the level of clinical significance regardless of which intervention was first presented. Second, when the participants were questioned as to which form of intervention they preferred, they indicated that they preferred CBT over exercise primarily because it was less effortful and required less pushing of oneself to engage in the activity. The study clearly showed that although there are effective methods of managing stress and depression, intervention effectiveness may not be sufficiently motivating to engage in the activity. This poses a problem for clinicians who wish to encourage secondarily traumatized clients to engage in exercise.

Bushman (2017) advocated criteria for the effective impact of exercise on stress disorders. The recommendation was to engage in moderate-intensity exercise 5 days per week for at least 30 min each day. Moderate-intensity exercise is defined as that which results in 60–80% of maximum heart rate. To determine maximum heart rate, one subtracts one's age from 220. This result is then multiplied by .60 or .80 (Motta, 2018). Let us take, for example, a 45-year-old psychotherapist who regularly treats traumatized clients 5 days a week and may be experiencing secondary trauma due to compassion fatigue. To calculate the heart rate that would be associated with moderate-intensity exercise, the following calculation would apply (220–45) × .6 (or .8) or 175 × .6 = 105 and 175 × .8 = 140. So, for moderate-intensity exercise, this therapist would have to maintain a heart rate of 105–140, and according to Bushman, do this for at least half an hour 5 times a week. This seems to be a demanding exercise schedule, and one wonders how practical this suggestion is. Therapists are often drained after treating clients all week and doing so week in and week out. The same is true for first responders and those enduring the emotional demands of caring for ill family members. It seems unlikely that any of these groups would take on what appears to be a demanding exercise schedule. Additionally, Bushman's exercise recommendation needs to be tempered by consideration of one's level of fitness, age, weight, and whether they are accustomed to exercising regularly. Rather than being presented as an absolute for attaining the stress-reducing benefits of exercise, it might be better to view any exercise as better than none.

From a clinical perspective, getting the client to exercise in any way would seem the most important hurdle rather than focusing on the amount or type of exercise that is to be done. As a result, it is probably best to start with an assessment of how much exercise the client is used to and then building from there. Whether the exercise is aerobic or non-aerobic is less important than whether the exercise program is manageable for the client. Available studies have focused a good deal on aerobic exercise, perhaps because it is more readily quantified than anaerobic exercise. When aerobic and anaerobic exercises are compared, there does not appear to be a distinct advantage of one over the other in terms of psychological benefits (e.g., Altchiler & Motta, 1997; Elkington et al., 2017). Further, it is often difficult to make a distinction between aerobic and non-aerobic as the latter will often give rise to elevated heart rates just as aerobic exercise does. It seems that the important question is which form of exercise is the client likely to do and not the specific types of that exercise. If the client does little to no exercise, then starting with perhaps a 10-min walk three times a week might be a reasonable beginning. Asking which exercise is best is somewhat like asking which form of relaxation is best. The answer is the one that the client is likely to do with regularity is the best. Regularity is more important than the specific characteristics of the exercise sessions (Motta, 2020).

## 9.5 Empirical Support for Exercise as a Secondary Trauma Intervention

Most of the empirical studies involving the therapeutic benefits of exercise focus on clinically oriented areas such as anxiety, depression, PTSD, OCD, and so on (Motta, 2018), and the exercise is often aerobic. It is not entirely clear why there are virtually no well-controlled comparison studies involving secondary traumatization per se and exercise (e.g., Bercier & Maynard, 2015), nor are there studies involving the use of anaerobic versus anaerobic exercise for treating secondary trauma. It appears likely that the reason for the scarcity of such studies may be because there are far fewer scales to assess secondary trauma in comparison to PTSD, anxiety, depression, and so on and similarly that anaerobic exercise is difficult to quantify when contrasted with aerobic exercise. For those reasons, the literature to be cited often deals with PTSD and comorbid emotional states such as anxiety and depression, and the exercise is primarily aerobic. This should not present a major problem if we are going to adhere to the stance taken by several authors (e.g., Figley, 1995; Figley, 2003; Harris, 1995; Jenkins & Baird, 2002) regarding the similarity of PTSD and STSD and the similarity of their treatment.

Shivakumar et al. (2017) recruited traumatized female veterans to determine whether exercise as a standalone intervention would be of benefit in reducing trauma reactions and depression. Depression is a common symptom in those who have been emotionally drained by secondary trauma experiences. The exercise was of aerobic nature but was graded in such a way that participants first engaged in brief and less intense exercise sessions and then worked their way up to brisk walking 30 to 40 min a day 4 days a week for 12 weeks. Prior to engaging in exercise, there was a brief stretching session. The completion rate of the 12-week program was 75% meaning that exercise program was readily tolerated. This dropout rate is like what is seen in those participating in yoga, meaning that the exercise was readily managed.

Study results showed significant reductions in measures of experienced trauma and depression and significant improvement on a measurement of quality of life. The authors report, "Finally, for patients with prominent avoidance related to their traumatic events, exercise may provide a safe and structured activity that can address social isolation and promote recovery" (p. 1813). This point regarding avoidance is of significance because individuals who are traumatized directly or indirectly, as in secondary traumatization, often manage their difficulties by active or subconscious avoidance of whatever was traumatizing to them. They tend to stay away from any therapeutic intervention that reminds them of their difficulties and stay away from the therapists who administer these treatments. Exercise does not come across as a formal therapeutic intervention, and because of this, at least in the Shivakumar et al. study, there was little avoidance as there was no dealing with specific aspects of their trauma other than completing paper-and-pencil measures.

The Shivakumar et al. (2017) study above involved a formal intervention in which traumatized individuals were prescribed a specific and controlled intervention of exercise to deal with trauma reactions. This intervention also had a positive impact on perceived quality of life. The question might be raised as to how effective is exercise when it is not prescribed? How well does exercise work in one's own environment when it is not put forward as an intervention but rather is engaged in voluntarily and as part of one's usual routines. Such a study was carried out by Whitworth et al. (2017).

In the Whitworth et al. (2017) study, an online longitudinal investigation was conducted whereby 182 participants completed measures of psychological distress, trauma reactions, sleep quality, alcohol usage, pain, and exercise behavior. The study found that there were significant reductions in all stress and related measures following voluntary strenuous exercise. The longer people engage in exercise and the more strenuous the exercise, the greater the benefit. The authors defined strenuous exercise as vigorous running or cycling. It is important to note that reductions were also found in measures of avoidance of dealing with one's psychological distress. Again, the relevance of this finding is that avoidance is a critical factor that prevents individuals from confronting, managing, and overcoming traumatizing issues and moving on with their lives. Whitworth et al. speculated that when one exercises vigorously, they become inured to physical distress because this helps facilitate continuance of exercise activity. The repeated practice of confronting the physical distress of exercise and the easing of the perceived exercise distress is then said to generalize to the handling psychological stressors in their lives. In this way a person becomes better able to manage stressors in general such as those that are typical of secondary trauma reactions. The findings of this study should not be interpreted as meaning that exercise must be intense for it to have various beneficial effects. Virtually all the literature in fact points in the opposite direction, that is, that moderate exercise is sufficient to produce emotional benefits.

An example of a study in which only moderately intense exercise was used was conducted by Diaz and Motta (2008). In this study adolescents who were between 14 and 17 years of age and who resided at a private residential treatment facility were previously screened for PTSD anxiety and depression and selected because of score elevations. The intervention involved 1 min of slow, leisurely walking as a warm-up, 23 min of moderate-intensity walking, and 1 min of slow walking as a cooldown. Clearly this was not an aerobically intense intervention, but it resulted in a significant reduction in PTSD-related symptoms that had evolved primarily from family discord, family disruptions, separations, and divorces. Reductions in anxiety and depression occurred, but these were less clear-cut than those in response to traumatic experiences. Many of the participants in this study had refused to participate in any form of structured psychotherapy at the treatment facility but seemed to take to and enjoy the exercise intervention.

The above study reveals that exercise need not be as intense as that highlighted in Whitworth et al. (2017) and that the impact of exercise, even moderate exercise, is applicable to adolescents as well as adults. In fact, exercise has beneficial effects on all ages including in children where it has been shown to also have a significant impact on cognitive functioning and judgment (Tomporowski et al., 2008) as well as psychological distress. Another study involving adolescents was conducted by Newman and Motta (2007) and involved a female-only sample at a residential treatment center. These young women had experienced a wide variety of traumatic experiences at home including family conflicts, physical and sexual abuse, maltreatment, or some combination of all of these. The form of exercise was varied to examine whether any specific form of exercise was more beneficial than others. The program ran for 8 weeks and involved 40-min sessions of exercise three times a week. The various exercises involved jogging, kickboxing, aerobic dancing, and so on, all of which produced and moderate aerobic effect of 60–80% of maximum heart rate. Results of the study showed significant reductions in anxiety, depression, and experienced trauma. A follow-up assessment was conducted 1 month after the exercise interventions, and treatment gains were maintained. There were no specific differences in outcome found when comparing the various forms of exercise, and it was concluded that exercise in general, rather than any specific form of exercise, was the important element in observed improvements. This finding was in accord with others that found that the specific form of exercise was not so important (e.g., Altchiler et al., 1997; Elkington et al., 2017).

A contributing factor that may have added to the beneficial impact of exercise in this group of adolescent females was that the exercises were done in groups and as the previous chapter has indicated, social support and contact can, in and of itself, have beneficial psychological effects as far as secondary traumatization is concerned. This study like the previous one that was presented pointed to two important conclusions. First, that exercise can be effective in reducing stress reactions not just in adults but also in young people. Second, the fact that this form of intervention requires not dealing with therapists, therapy, or addressing unpleasant issues related to traumatic experiences makes it a useful and easily accessible intervention for those who have no desire to commit to formal treatment or to deal with troubling psychological issues. If secondarily traumatized participants are willing to address their difficulties directly in formal counseling, the available empirical research suggests that exercise may provide additional psychological benefits given its stress-reducing and mood-elevating characteristics.

## 9.6 Summary

Exercise has been shown to be a stress reliever that enhances mood states and increases perceptions of well-being. For this reason, it is put forward as a viable form of intervention for those suffering from secondary trauma, regardless of its source. Exercise appears to reduce distress in and of itself but can also be considered as a therapeutic adjunct to more traditional forms of counseling. There is no general agreement as to why exercise has such beneficial effects and several hypotheses have been offered. Some of these hypotheses are physiological and suggest that alterations in brain chemistry or temperature are what produce the benefit. Other hypotheses emphasize more psychological factors such as distraction or the enhancement of self-efficacy perceptions. The bodymind position of Candace Pert suggests that body and mind are not separable, and if one adheres to this position then the search for the *why* of exercise benefits seems not to be fruitful.

Several research studies are highlighted that clearly show that exercise in and of itself can significantly reduce trauma reactions along with depression and anxiety, while also enhancing perceptions of well-being. One of the real benefits of exercise in comparison to traditional psychotherapy is that it does not require the direct confronting of trauma-related issues. Such confronting often produces a level of anxiety that results in avoidance of therapy and therapists. Studies were presented in which adolescents who had suffered from experiencing family difficulties not only psychologically benefited from exercise but preferred it to traditional therapy. The same was found with an adult sample suffering from depression. Overall, exercise is a valuable tool for dealing with secondary traumatization and comorbid conditions of anxiety and depression, regardless of the specific nature or source of the traumatic experience. A potential drawback of exercise, as was shown in the Mulcahy (1988) study, is that for participants who are willing to deal directly with their stressors in therapy, exercise is seen as more effortful and therefore less desirable than traditional forms of counseling. Nevertheless, available research points to the significant potential benefit of exercise for those who have experienced various forms of trauma including secondary trauma.

# Chapter 10
# Mindfulness Meditation and Secondary Trauma

Mindfulness meditation is effective in reducing symptoms related to burnout or secondary traumatization and increasing one's perceptions of satisfaction with caregiver work (e.g., Germer, 2005). The latter is referred to as compassion satisfaction (e.g., Ash et al., 2021; Stamm, 2010) and is relevant to the feelings of self-fulfillment and positive self-perception evolving from having played a role in helping others. In contrast, the emotional exhaustion and burnout that commonly occur in response to meeting the needs of others who have been traumatized often call for some type of self-care intervention such as mindfulness meditation. Maslach and Leiter (1997) claim that burnout from job demands can result in emotional depletion to such a degree that there is an erosion of one's dignity and spirit. This erosion is often seen in those experiencing secondary trauma.

While mindfulness can be beneficial in ameliorating the effects of secondary traumatization, it is not an "easy" intervention to become proficient in. Popular media makes it seem like mindful states are readily attainable. "From classrooms to corporations, mindfulness is being practiced by a wide array of people—at times being marketed as a quick-fix solution to stress" (Treleaven, 2018, p. 25). In 2018 Treleaven indicated that a Google search revealed almost 20 thousand applications for which mindfulness would be helpful. However, there appears to be a large gulf between popularity and quick fixes and "real-world" implementation.

## 10.1 Challenges in Using Mindfulness to Address Secondary Trauma

Despite its effectiveness, if one expects mindfulness to have enduring utility, then it must be practiced regularly, and, in that regard, it is somewhat like exercise. One does not simply do exercise for a little while and expect it to have long-term benefits in reducing secondary trauma. It must be practiced regularly, and this is also true

© The Author(s), under exclusive license to Springer Nature Switzerland AG 2023

R. W. Motta, *Secondary Trauma*, https://doi.org/10.1007/978-3-031-44308-4_10

with mindfulness practice. Those expecting to benefit from mindfulness meditation should expect to make it regular activity in their lives. Ash et al. (2021) found beneficial effects of using compassion meditation in a study involving those who are involved in hospital chaplaincy work and who experience secondary trauma by way of compassion fatigue. However, the effects of feeling less depressed, less anxious, and being satisfied with one's work following mediative practice were not maintained in a 4-month follow-up period after meditation practice was no longer required. This negative outcome supported the need for ongoing practice of meditation to maintain its effectiveness. One realizes at the outset that meditation requires a commitment in that it must become an ongoing routine involving daily practice.

Another caveat when considering the valuable tool of mindfulness meditation in alleviating secondary trauma and enhancing compassion satisfaction is that in addition to the need for ongoing practice, mindfulness meditation is not easy. Meditation typically involves focusing of attention, but this is difficult because, "In many ways, the mind has a mind of its own, moving as it does from one thought to the next with little input from the thinker" (Motta, 2020, p. 67). These mind wanderings, or to use a term attributed to William James, *stream of consciousness* (Editors of *Encyclopedia Britannica,* n.d.), are something of a tyranny of our thinking processes in that they usually occur without our intending or wanting them. The mind wanders through a process of association, whereby one thought, regardless of how tangential or trivial, leads to a related thought and that to another associated thought. It is difficult to stop this process without focused effort. When one observes their thinking, one sees a disconnected and automatic process of mind wandering that appears to be taking place, all on its own with little input from us. "Studies have shown these places [mind wanderings] are usually in the past or the future: you may ponder recent events or distant, strong memories; you may dread upcoming events or eagerly anticipate them … What you're generally *not* doing when your mind is wandering is directly experiencing the present moment" (Wright, 2017, p. 46).

A typical goal of meditation is directed attention as a counter to the normal, random wanderings of the mind. "Mindfulness means paying attention in a particular way: on purpose, in the present moment, and non-judgmentally" (Kabat-Zinn, 1994, p. 4). So, for example, the person involved in meditation might direct their focus to their breathing and note the rising and falling of their diaphragm. They might note the sensation of the air passing through their nostrils. When mind wandering occurs, as it inevitably will, they might redirect their focus back to their breathing or perhaps direct it elsewhere such as to the sensations in their body. How are their feet feeling while planted on the floor? How are their legs and buttocks feeling? Are there any aches and pains in any part of the body? One might engage in a systematic and detailed survey of the sensations in the body using a technique called "body scan" (Kabat-Zinn, 2005, pp. 250–253), where attention is given to the sensations of specific body parts, for example, the right big toe, and then to successive body parts. All these activities are intended to stop mind wandering and direct one's focus to what is happening now, at this moment. How is this or that area of the body feeling at this specific time? What thoughts have you observed running through your mind? The goal here is to observe the thoughts and let them pass, rather than pursuing them or letting them stimulate related thoughts. A further goal is to gain control over the mind to focus it while also accepting the fact that the mind's nature is to wander, so there is no need to become self-critical, frustrated, or judgmental about how one's mind is operating.

Horn et al. (2014) have referred to the content of the automatic state of mind wandering as *the default mode network*. When one is engaged in unfocused mental activity, the mind wanders to the future or the past, and this network, when observed on brain scans, reveals interconnections among the medial prefrontal cortex, posterior cingulate cortex, and amygdala, which is associated with fear reactions. Thus, our thoughts are often emotionally driven. We may like to believe that we have ultimate control over our thoughts, but it appears that, most of the time, the brain is operating independently and flitting from one thought to the next without our input. With ongoing practice, one becomes increasingly able to limit mind wandering, but it is highly unlikely that one will ever be able to stop mind wandering in a typical meditative practice session, which often lasts 20 min to one half hour.

Another view that might help explain why the mind wanders is that of Damasio (2010). Damasio reports that the brain is composed of approximately 90 billion interconnected neurons, and many of these interconnections form semiautonomous modules. There are modules for past events, future events, desires, aspirations, worries, and many more. A small segment of the brain's activity underlies awareness. In contrast, most of the brain's activity is taken up by regulating unconscious functions such as respiration, temperature regulation, movement activities, and others. The modules are said to compete for a place on the comparatively small stage of awareness. When one of the modules is not focused on and not pursued as occurs during meditation, where one does not follow or pursue one's thoughts, another module attempts to take its place. This may be one interpretation of our ceaseless mind wandering. It is the replacement of one module's presence on the stage of awareness by another module that seeks to take its place. And so, it seems that when we try not to focus on a specific preoccupation, another readily replaces it, and we experience this automatic replacement process as mind wandering.

## 10.2 Why Would Mindfulness Be Beneficial in Managing Secondary Trauma

Secondary trauma reactions generally refer to negative psychological states that evolve from the immersion in, and commitment to, helping others and/or to being negatively impacted by the emotional distress of others. This immersion sets up a tendency to obsess over and ruminate about the other's difficulties. It becomes difficult to break away from these consuming thoughts. They often become a part of the traumatized individual's default mode network. Meditation is a willful gaining of control over one's thoughts so that the current of rumination and dwelling over distressing situations is reduced and is directed to the here and now. "Meditation means learning how to get out this current, sit by the bank and listen to it, learn from it, and then use its energies to guide us rather than tyrannize us" (Kabat-Zinn, 1994, p. 9). So, one of the benefits that meditation can have in managing secondary trauma is to gain control over and cease, or at least decrease, the stream of negative obsessions and ruminations.

In addition to impeding negative thoughts and ruminations, there are also positive outcomes of meditation such as the enhancement of compassion satisfaction (Stamm, 2010) and others that are difficult to define. Germer (2005) points out that "Mindfulness has to be experienced to be known" (p. 8). Like love, mindfulness is better experienced to understand it rather than using words to describe it. Because mindfulness involves nonjudgmental acceptance of situations, people, and all else within the sphere of awareness and experience, this nonjudgmental stance spreads to one's view of oneself and others. Mindfulness brings on a noncritical, nonjudgmental acceptance of the way things are and the way we are. This stance, if fully accepted and incorporated into one's worldview, can be tremendously stress relieving. The person who is experienced in the practice of mindfulness accepts things as they are and spends far less time being consumed over how things "should" be or how "I should be." Mindfulness purportedly enhances self-regulation in three ways: "The regulation of attention, body awareness, and emotional regulation" (Treleaven, 2018, p. 31). Regulation and control are contrasted with, and the antithesis of, perceptions of being out of control of one's environment and out of control of one's felt experience as commonly occurs in secondary trauma.

## 10.3 Brief History of Mindfulness

The word *mindfulness* is derived from the Latin word *meditatum*, which is said to be translatable as the word "ponder" (Mead, 2020). Mindfulness is a translation of the Pali word *sati*, which implies attention, awareness, and remembering (Motta, 2020). Pali, a language closely related to Sanskrit, was used to convey the teachings of the Buddha (Siddhartha Gautama) who is said to have attained enlightenment around the time of 500 BCE. Buddhist practices and teachings at that time were focused on the development of an understanding of the relatedness of all things rather than attempting to understand the mind of God. Thus, meditative practices as engaged in today are more oriented toward the development of awareness than toward any religious focus. Some writers (e.g., Dienstmann, 2018) suggest that meditation may have a history that dates back even further than Buddhist teachings, to around five thousand years ago.

Despite its seeming nonreligious origins, a great many of the world's religions incorporate some form of mindful attention to better understand God's works. Thus, Christianity, Judaism, Sikhism, Taoism, and many others use meditation as a tool to deepen faith and this tool can be acquired in different ways. The use of or "saying of" the rosary, for example, involves a focus of attention as one repeats a prayer for each of the rosary beads. A decade is represented by five sets of ten beads, with each set separated by a larger bead. A five-decade version would have 59 beads. Those sets used by nuns might cover 15 decades. Usually, the same prayer is stated in one's mind for each of the ten beads, and a different one is used for the larger bead. One can see how repeating the same prayer numerous times requires a considerable degree of focused attention, and this is a central feature of meditation. Islamic tradition involves the saying of God's name numerous times along with specific rituals involving controlled breathing (Ginsburgh, 2006). The goal here is to focus one's attention to get closer to God. But, as stated above, mindfulness meditation as it is practiced in the West today is generally not religiously oriented. Rather it emphasizes focused attention, nonjudgmental awareness of oneself and others, and the ability to be "in the present moment" without being distracted by endless chains of associated thoughts and preoccupations with the past or with future expectations.

## 10.4 Mindfulness as a Therapeutic Tool

Considerations of the role of mindfulness in psychotherapy and medicine can be traced to the era of Sigmund Freud who wrote about the oceanic feelings associated with mindfulness but also derided it as a "regressive experience" (Motta, 2020, p. 68). Other well-known theorists took a less negative stance and wrote of the potential usefulness of mindfulness within the therapeutic context, for example, Horney, Fromm, and Jung. In more recent times, the popular musical group, *The Beatles*, sang of meditative and psychedelic experiences, and this helped spread a positive of meditation among young people. Herbert Benson, a Harvard Medical School-affiliated cardiologist, developed an interest in meditative practices but to avoid potential negative feedback in writing about such a seemingly "unscientific" process used the term relaxation instead of meditation. His book *The Relaxation Response* (1975) elaborated upon relaxation (meditation) practices that could help in reducing heart disease because of its stress-neutralizing characteristics. Another popularizer was Ram Dass (born Richard Alpert) at Harvard who wrote a wildly popular book, *Be Here Now* (1978), which sold over a million copies. The book's emphasis was on the importance of being aware of and living in the present as an alternative to being consumed by ruminations involving the past or the hopes, fears, and expectations of the future.

A major popularizer and prominent spokesperson for mindfulness meditation in the USA has been Jon Kabat-Zinn. His training was in molecular biology, but while studying at the Massachusetts Institute of Technology, he developed a consuming interest in mindfulness practices. Following the obtaining of his doctorate, he formed a stress reduction clinic at the University of Massachusetts in 1979 where he received referrals of medical patients who were often experiencing intractable pain from often fatal illnesses and for whom there were few options for further pain reduction. While there he also trained physicians in the application of his mindfulness-based stress reduction (MBSR) procedures at his MBSR clinic. A typical course of MBSR in which both patients and staff participated involved 45-min daily sessions of mindfulness practice for a period of 8 weeks. Kabat-Zinn went on to form the *Center for Mindfulness in Medicine, Health Care, and Society* at the

University of Massachusetts Medical School for the training of physicians and treatment of patients (Center for Mindfulness, Health Care, and Society, n.d.). He subsequently produced a series of popular books, including *Full Catastrophe Living: Using the Wisdom of Your Body and Mind to Face Stress, Pain, and Illness* (1990), *Wherever You Go, There You Are: Mindfulness Meditation in Everyday Life* (1994), and *Coming to Our Senses: Healing Ourselves and the World Through Mindfulness* (2005). His workshops, other books, TV appearances, apps, and so on have also contributed to the acceptance of mindfulness as a stress-reducing and awareness-enhancing activity.

Mindfulness meditation has become such an integral part of psychological treatments that it is a component of several CBT therapies. Some of these include acceptance and commitment therapy (ACT) (Hayes et al., 2016), dialectical behavior therapy (DBT) (Linehan, 1993), and mindfulness-based cognitive therapy (MBCT) (Teasdale et al., 2000). Given that all of these psychotherapeutic methods are empirically supported treatments (ESTs), it can be reasonably asserted that mindfulness practices represent empirically validated treatments (Hayes et al., 2004). However, it is important to consider the following. In most instances, formal CBT or CBT with a mindfulness component will not be necessary in managing most secondary trauma cases. Rather, mindfulness meditation is presented here as a self-care strategy for those whose work or personal experiences have left them secondarily traumatized.

It has been the position of this book that secondary trauma and primary trauma experiences such as PTSD are different phenomena despite some degree of overlap. This overlap occurs in cases of extreme secondary traumatization whereby the sufferer may show many of the symptoms of PTSD. In those cases, CBT may be called for, or other forms of alternative therapies might be used (e.g., Motta, 2020). Mindfulness meditation for secondary trauma is presented here as a self-care strategy which, along with other such strategies like exercise and social support, can be implemented without engaging in formal individual or group psychotherapy. As a rule, secondary trauma evolves from giving to others and acquiring their emotional distress responses. The secondarily traumatized individual is often emotionally drained. PTSD, or primary traumatization, is usually the outcome of experiencing extreme fear and often a threat to one's life. Secondary trauma often leaves sufferers emotionally overwrought and exhausted. Primary trauma produces prolonged fear responses, alteration of self-view, and distrust of an environment that is seen as threatening and needing to be avoided.

## 10.5 Specific Benefits of Mindfulness Practice

Turlow (2017, pp. 4–5) describes the benefits that can accrue with regular practice of mindfulness meditation. What is presented here is how mindfulness might be of value in managing secondary trauma based on Turlow's views. These benefits include the following:

*Emotional tolerance and flexibility.* While secondary trauma may evoke feelings of anxiety, depression, and anger, we learn that these are temporary, and we gain confidence that we can navigate through them.

*Enhanced relaxation.* One of the ways that relaxation is enhanced is by a reduction of the ruminative preoccupations that typically occur in secondary trauma. Rather than obsessively focusing on these disturbing thoughts, one focuses on body sensations, breathing, and so on, all of which pull one away from negative rumination.

*Reduction of automatic reactions.* With mindfulness we develop a greater perspective and with this an increased ability to choose how we react rather than reacting reflexively.

*Increased attentional control.* By attending to where the mind goes in its default network meanderings, we can change our patterns of attention so that we reduce the focus on past secondary traumatic experiences and future expectations.

*The cultivation of self-compassion.* With mindfulness practice we learn that some of the negativism, cynicism, and rumination that accompany secondary traumatization are to be expected. In this way we gain a greater capacity to accept ourselves and to adopt an attitude of kindness, forgiveness, and compassion to ourselves as well as others.

*Reduction of avoidance.* Avoidance of painful memories and feelings is a common response to traumatic experiences. While avoidance may work in alleviating pain in the near term, it prolongs distress in the long run. Mindfulness facilitates being present with our experiences including those that are painful. With practice we develop a calmer and more accepting approach to difficult feelings and thoughts.

*Reduction of self-judgment.* Those who experience primary trauma such as seen in PTSD often have a negativistic sense of self. This is because they have encountered a level of fear that causes them to react like a "frightened animal." Many feel animalized or dehumanized. In a similar way, those who are secondarily traumatized may feel they have failed to do all they could to help others and as a result may become self-critical. They might also acquire a negative sense of self that is like that of the primarily traumatized person perhaps because of a close and extended relationship with that person. Either way, mindfulness, if practiced diligently, emphasizes acceptance and a nonjudgmental stance, including a nonjudgmental perspective of oneself.

*Making this moment bigger.* Mindfulness helps in not getting overly caught up in one's immediate discomfort and pain. "If we can broaden our experience of this moment a bit in a positive way, it can feel easier to handle our past suffering and worries about the future" (Turlow, 2017, p. 5). A focus on the present moment is a central component of mindfulness practice.

*Cultivating a balanced perspective.* Secondarily traumatized people may distance themselves from their bodily sensations. For that reason, one sees an elevation of drinking and drug use (e.g., Brooks et al., 2016; Mitchell, 2011) to deaden pain. Meditation helps one develop a more balanced perspective by integrating the body sensations and awareness. Mindfulness also helps us become less submerged in and encompassed by pain. The person skilled in the use of mindfulness can see that they are not defined by pain but rather that pain is external to them.

*Re-perceiving ourselves and the world.* Secondarily traumatized individuals tend to be stuck in a mindset that convinces them that traumatizing situations will continue without change. With meditative practice we learn to adjust our mindset to find new possibilities for coping with difficult situations. Mindfulness facilitates the capability of distancing and observing situations from an objective standpoint. When this is done, new possibilities and potential for change often present themselves.

## 10.6 General Guidelines for Mindfulness Practice

The typical view of meditation is that of sitting in a lotus position with the spine erect and eyes closed. However, the practice of mindfulness can be engaged in anywhere and in any manner including standing, lying down, sitting, and even walking. If lying down, one might choose the corpse pose with the back flat on the floor, arms slightly away from the body with palms facing upward, heels on the floor, and legs slightly separated. If sitting, a zafu or meditation cushion might be used as a pillow under the buttocks, with the legs crossed, palms facing upward, and resting on the knees. A straight-back chair can also be used with palms on one's knees or facing upward. In walking meditation, one focuses on the slow progress of one foot in front of the other while attending to where the heel gently touches the ground and how the body moves its weight forward toward the ball of the foot. Attention is paid not to wandering thoughts but to how the feet, legs, and body move and how they feel as one moves forward.

If there is any commonality in these methods, or any other method of meditating, it is attentional focus. One focuses on one's current physical and mental state or a specific concept or image and tries not to be pulled along by random wandering thoughts. It has been only half-jokingly said that one can meditate while emptying the dishwasher just so long as the attention is focused on such as activities as removal of plates, cups, utensils, and so on, how they are lifted, where they are placed, and how they feel. Again, the commonality among these various approaches is mental focus on current happenings and not allowing the mind to drift aimlessly from one thought to the next.

Other "how-to" issues in mindfulness practice are attitude and when practice takes place. An attitude of acceptance is of central importance. One must accept that their thoughts will drift and there is a need to bring them back without negative self-evaluation. Being self-critical in evaluating one's "success" in meditating defeats the purpose of striving for a nonjudgmental stance toward oneself and others. The time of day when one meditates is not laid out in stone, but it is typically done in the mornings for two reasons. First, by engaging in meditation early, one prioritizes it as an important aspect of their life. Second, by doing so one is less likely to get caught up in daily concerns and activities and is thereby less vulnerable to being pulled away by distractions.

When asked how much time is needed to meditate, Kabat-Zinn (1994) honestly remarked, “How should I know?” (1994, p. 121). In this offhanded remark, he was implying that there are many factors that determine how long a meditation session should last including the free time available, the practitioner’s ability to focus, the nature of that day’s demands, and other factors. In his work at the University of Massachusetts Medical Center, his mindfulness-based stress reduction sessions typically ran for 45 min. More commonly, meditation is practiced for approximately 20 min daily. Soler et al. (2014), in a study of mindfulness practices, found that the amount of time one spends during each session of mindfulness meditation is less important than the regularity of making meditation a daily practice on virtually all days. While the specifics of what posture to assume, what to focus on, what time of day, and how long one practices are all variable, the regularity of practice is somewhat more important. To reap the benefits of mindfulness meditation, regular daily practice is critical. Like exercise, one attains the most benefits less so from the specific type of exercise than whether it is done as a life routine. Routine practice of mindfulness results in the greatest self-reported benefits (Soler et al., 2014).

## 10.7 Specific Steps in Mindfulness Practice

1. Strive for an attentive and comfortable orientation whether sitting, lying down, or walking. If sitting, establish an erect and dignified position. If lying down, the face, palms, and feet are often directed upward. If walking, a slow, rhythmic, and careful placement of one foot in front of the other is engaged in with attention of what part of the foot is making contact.
2. Eyes are closed or half open and oriented to a place 2 to 3 feet away. The eyes are typically not focused but simply oriented in a direction if open. The “gaze” of one’s open or closed eyes is inward. This is even the case in walking meditation where the focus is not on where one is headed but rather on sensations, movement, and body positions.
3. A critical issue is attentional focus. One might typically begin with a focus on one’s breathing and becoming aware of the air passing into and out of one’s nostrils or of the diaphragm slowly moving inward and outward. One might also have a specific physical target or concept to focus on. But again, the critical issue is to maintain focal attention while also accepting that doing so will be difficult and that the mind is likely to wander and that this is to be expected. When the mind does wander, the specific thoughts are not pursued but are simply let go, and the attention is brought back to the initial point of focus.
4. Once one gains an increasing ability to attend, the focus can be redirected to other occurrences such as the sounds of traffic, the wind, the sounds of birds, the ringing in one’s ears, the flow of one’s thoughts, and how long it takes for one to

catch oneself in their mind wanderings. Awareness of the present moment is the difficult goal that one is attempting to attain.
5. Become aware of your motivations for ending the mindfulness session. In doing so we become more self-aware of what it is that is pulling us along. What is tyrannizing us and making us something of an automaton, and who is pulled along by their wandering thoughts? This inner awareness and realization that we, and everyone else, are somewhat at the mercy of our thoughts can lead to a greater appreciation and nonjudgmental acceptance of oneself and others.
6. Practice daily or as regularly as possible. Give mindfulness meditation priority so it can broaden and deepen your life and help the secondarily traumatized individual be better able to cope with and manage their daily stressors.

## 10.8 A Sampling of Meditations Relevant to Secondary Trauma

The general practice of mindfulness and attending to body sensations, breathing, environmental sounds, and so on has been shown empirically to be effective in ameliorating symptoms of secondary trauma (e.g., Whitebird et al., 2012). However, after having attained some degree of stability and tranquility through general meditative practice, one might begin engaging in specific kinds of meditations that are oriented toward the unique profile of difficulties of the secondary trauma sufferer.

## 10.9 Loving-Kindness Meditation

Kabat-Zinn (1994) reports that the Dali Lama, when asked about his beliefs, stated "My religion is kindness" (p. 168) and with this in mind, the loving-kindness meditation is appropriate particularly for those traumatized individuals who lack self-compassion. The goal of the loving-kindness meditation is to give kindness and love to oneself and others. Recall that the secondarily traumatized person is essentially hurt by the hurt of others. These people often feel drained and demoralized and that they have not successfully met the needs of others or the demands placed on them. As a result, they may ruminate over their perceived failings and shortcomings. In the loving-kindness meditation, one might repeat a certain self-compassionate series of verbalizations (Salzberg, 1995). These verbalizations can be similar to "May I be safe. May I be happy. May I have peace. May I be healthy. May I have tranquility. May I actions be kind" (Motta, 2020, p. 79).

This specific meditation not only supplants the automatic, self-critical ruminations commonly seen in those experiencing secondary trauma, but it also provides tranquility and emotional sustenance to those who have given so much of themselves. Once the individual begins to develop a greater sense of harmony and tranquility, they may then imaginably share this meditation by offering it to specific family members and others with whom they are close. And once they are comfortable with this, they might then imaginably send loving wishes to those with whom they have conflict or whom they don't particularly like. In wishing positive experiences for those who are disliked, the meditator is showing and developing the quality of nonjudgment. The loving-kindness meditation can eventually include nonhuman entities or the earth itself as a life-giving and nurturing entity. At this stage in the loving-kindness meditation, there is an appreciation of the fact that we and those with whom we are acquainted, as well as other entities living and nonliving, are interconnected and interdependent. Acceptance and kindness are given to all in the loving-kindness meditation in a manner of the Dali Lama whose "religion is kindness."

## 10.10 Everest Meditation

The Everest meditation is derived from Kabat-Zinn's Mountain Meditation (1994, pp. 135–140). The top of Mount Everest is on the Nepal-China border and at 29,035 feet is the highest mountain in the world. It was first climbed on May 29, 1953, by New Zealander Edmund Hillary and Sherpa Tenzing Norgay. Their success was preceded by numerous failed attempts owning to horrendous weather conditions that are marked by winds that at times exceed 200 miles per hour in sub-zero blizzard conditions. Everest is the ultimate prize of professional climbers and nonprofessionals, many of whom have died in their efforts to reach its peak. The Tibetan name for Everest is Chomolungma—Goddess Mother of Mountains.

The mystique and majesty of Everest can make it a useful focus of meditation practice. Kabat-Zinn (1994) suggests a sitting meditation where one imagines oneself as the mountain itself. The buttocks are imagined to be the rock base and foundation of this massive peak. The head is envisioned as its peak with shoulders and arms as its various outcroppings. The mountain is immobile, impenetrable, and unchangeable. Its weather can range from howling blizzards or mild conditions. It is bathed in chilling darkness or climatically mild, brilliant sunshine. It is visited by thousands yearly and numerous climbers attempt to summit its peak, but most fail to do so. Death is common on Everest due to falls, hypothermia, pulmonary edema, anoxia, and other calamities. Despite the vicious weather conditions, the blasting winds, the hordes of ambitious climbers striving for glory, the unfortunate calamities, and deaths, the mountain is unchanged, solid, and impenetrable. It bears all assaults and efforts to summit its peak with quiet and stable equanimity. And it is this stability, this impenetrability, and this ability to handle all that the sitting meditator attempts to identify with. In seeing oneself as Everest, the person engaged in sitting meditation sees themselves as equally strong and imperturbable.

The secondarily traumatized person is often stressed, exhausted, emotionally drained, depressed, cynical, and anxious. Everest is none of these. It is unphased by any human assault upon it or by the vicious weather conditions that it regularly encounters. The secondarily traumatized meditator attempts to incorporate these characteristics. Whereas they may feel overwhelmed and exhibit compassion fatigue due to the excessive demands that are placed upon them, Everest experiences none of this. Everest has remained unchanged in the past and will be unchanged in the future. This image is incorporated into the self of the traumatized person who is meditating.

One sits quietly, crossed-legged, and abandons all thoughts and burdens that they have brought with them. They envision themselves as strong as Everest. Able to withstand the emotional demands and even potential assaults that are inherent in their work as frontline workers, health providers, or family members caring for those in need of what they can provide. They sit with this image of impenetrability for 20 to 30 min, only to return to it the next day and the next. With time and practice, they hopefully begin to acquire the strength of Everest which, as the highest mountain on earth, is the essence of strength and endurance. Similar mountains or imperturbable objects can be used in meditations such as this one, but Everest has a unique mystique and is associated with the essence of strength and permanence. With time and practice, the secondarily traumatized meditator can become strengthened and feel less vulnerable to, and less impacted by, the emotionally depleting demands that are placed upon them. The Everest meditation can become a valuable tool resource for those who need relief from their stressors.

## 10.11 The Quiet Pond

In the woods, away from the sounds of traffic and the buzzing activities of humanity, there lies a quiet pond. The pond is not readily seen by the random hiker as it is not near any trails and is surrounded by a thick forest and hidden by a dense aggregation of fir trees. This pond is about a quarter mile across and is no more than 12 feet at its deepest point. The pond supports a variety of fish, insects, and plant life. Its shallowness allows sunlight to penetrate its depth and thereby support plant life even at its deepest point.

This hidden pond, because it is most often shielded from the winds typically has a mirror-like surface. It is still, quiet, and serene and is in harmony with its environment and reflects that environment. It, along with the surrounding trees, makes for a tranquil and naturally beautiful ecosystem. The pond sits in stillness and despite the occasional sounds of insects is the very essence of tranquility, peace, and harmony. If its surface is disturbed in any way, it returns to stillness. If a fish jumps to capture an insect on the surface, the rippling of the surface subsides and returns to mirror-like stillness. If anything falls into the pond, it either floats on the surface or sinks to the bottom, but in either case, the pond returns to tranquility, stillness, and serenity. Its mirror-like surface is not like the mirrors we know that can shatter or crack. Nothing shatters or cracks the pond's surface. Regardless of what takes place on that surface, it eventually returns to utter flatness and reflects the trees, clouds, and sky that shine up from its surface.

The person enduring the daily stresses that commonly eventuate in secondary traumatization can use the pond meditation to help quiet the stressors placed upon them. They either sit in an erect position on a chair or zafu, or they might engage in this meditation lying down with their back pressed against and fully supported by the floor. In these positions one imagines that they are the quiet pond. With practice, their emotional state becomes tranquil, quiet, serene, and nourishing just as the pond is serene and provides a nourishing environment that supports animal and plant life. And, just like the pond, when a disturbing event takes place, stillness and quiet are soon restored. The natural state of the pond is one of stillness and quiet, and this becomes the natural state of the person engaged in purposeful and repeated meditation of the quiet pond. In their meditation one imagines that they are that pond and that they can return to tranquility, peace, and lack of upset, just as the pond does. Regardless of what is happening in the world of human conflicts, natural disasters, economic crises, political storms, or any other event, the pond and the person who has acquired the characteristics of the pond return to stillness and quiet. Their emotions and nervous systems return to the quiet and mirror-like tranquility of the pond. Kabat-Zinn (1994) offers a similar meditation, "The Lake Meditation" (p. 141) for those who are troubled or traumatized or for those who simply wish to attain greater tranquility and acceptance in their lives.

Meditations involving specific imagery such as the loving-kindness meditation, the Everest meditation, and the pond meditation can provide an important resource for those who are distressed by the travails of others. These shared traumas are ubiquitous, and their routine and repeated nature can be depleting. It is not necessary to imagine specific meditations that provide love, strength, and peace. The very practice of mindfulness—that is, being in the present moment and not being dragged about by preoccupations and concerns that impinge on one's consciousness—can in and of itself bring about the relief from stress and the return to equanimity that is so beneficial for one's functioning. The imagery meditations are simply presented as a tool for those who might find specific meditations preferential to the more general sitting in stillness in the present moment.

## 10.12 Empirical Backing

Alternative interventions, such as meditation, yoga, and exercise, have empirical support for their use in managing trauma including secondary traumatization. The level of support might not be as substantial as that found for traditional therapies such as CBT, and from this it could be argued that they are less effective, but it is more likely that because they are not considered to be mainstream scientific topics, researchers are not as inclined to investigate them nor are abundant sources of funding available for their study. Nevertheless, the empirical support for meditative practices as means of coping with traumatic experience is substantial.

In a review of 12 mindfulness meditation studies (Banks et al., 2015), it was concluded that these types of interventions can be effective in reducing various trauma symptoms, especially avoidance. Avoidance is a particularly vexing characteristic of those who have been traumatized and involves a tendency to stay away from anything, including thoughts, images, emotions, or behaviors that remind sufferers of their traumatizing experiences. Avoidance may be helpful in the short run as it reduces the immediate aversive impact of anxiety, but unfortunately not dealing with trauma symptoms lessens the probability of overcoming one's difficulties. Hilton et al. (2017) found that mindfulness-based stress reduction (MBSR), yoga, and the use of mantra repetitions were effective in reducing trauma-like symptoms in comparison to treatment as usual (TAU). In another study involving a review of the literature (Kim et al., 2013), it was found that 12 of the 16 studies that were reviewed showed a positive impact of meditation on trauma-related symptoms. Similarly, a review by Vujanovic et al. (2013) showed meditation to be more effective than TAU, attention-matched controls, and active controls in terms of amelioration of trauma-related symptoms.

Ash et al. (2021) evaluated a cognitively based compassion training (CBCT), which was a group-delivered meditation intervention for hospital chaplain residents ($n = 15$). The chaplain residents are expected to provide emotional and spiritual support to hospitalized patients and as a result are exposed to potentially secondary traumatic experiences. Chaplain residents who were assigned to the CBCT group showed decreases in burnout and anxiety when compared to a matched waitlist control group but were not found to significantly differ from the control group on a measure of compassion satisfaction. While the results of the study were in the expected direction of lessening secondary trauma-related symptoms, these benefits were found to fade after a 4-month follow-up. What the study highlights is the need for continued meditation practice to have appreciable and sustained benefits.

It would appear from this study and others that mindfulness meditation and other forms of meditative practice must be ongoing for at least the duration of time that individuals are exposed to potentially secondarily traumatizing environments for the meditative practice to have a meaningful impact. When meditation interventions emphasize self-compassion, as well as compassion for others, significant positive correlations are found with life satisfaction and happiness and significant negative correlations with depressive rumination, anxiety, and negativistic perfectionism (e.g., Neff et al., 2007; Odou & Brinker, 2014). Thus, the benefits of mindfulness meditation and other forms of meditative practice not only function to protect against the negative impact of secondary traumatization but also function to enhance happiness and life satisfaction in general. Again, regular and dedicated practices appear to be essential in obtaining these benefits.

## 10.13 Case Presentation

John came into therapy because he was experiencing anxieties arising from a newly established romantic relationship. The woman he was seeing appears to have been sexually assaulted by her stepfather on multiple occasions. Her relating of these experiences to John resulted in high levels of anxiety for him because it triggered memories of his own traumatic past. Her trauma was reactivating his. In reviewing his history, John reported that he did not feel that his parents should have had a child because they seemed ill-equipped to serve as models of normal behavior, nor were they able to provide a consistently nurturant emotional climate in the home. John's memory of his childhood was one of physical abuse, but he claimed that the emotional abuse that he received was even worse than the physical. As a child his mother would slap him and pull his hair over what she saw as his laziness in cleaning the dishes, keeping his room neat and tidy, or not spending enough time on his schoolwork. Her disappointment in "my numerous failings" was a constant theme with this mother. His father's abuse involved punches in the face and stomach and being whipped with a thick leather belt. What was most disturbing to John was that these physical assaults were unpredictable. He could not discern when his mother would see his room or the dishes as meeting her standards of neatness or cleanliness, nor could he determine when his father would take offense at something he might have said that would then result in his being pummeled. But again, John stated that the emotional abuse was even more damaging than the physical.

What he recalls is that his father felt John was weak and "not a man." His father would make comments like, "Why don't you put on a dress, you little faggot?" John described himself as introverted and shy, and these traits must have triggered his father into seeing John as unmanly. John stated that he believed that his demeanor angered his father and that he might have believed that beating John would "toughen me up." John found his mother's behavior more difficult to comprehend. At times she was overly close and "almost seductive." When John had nightmares, which were common, she would have him sleep in bed with her and her husband. She would be scantily clad and would "spoon" with John in a way that seemed inappropriate and uncomfortable to him. However, most of the time she was remote and castigating. She often referred to John as "my idiot son" and continuously communicated her overall disappointment in him and his general incompetence in most things. This seemed to be her rationale for the slapping and hair pulling. John described his childhood and early adolescence as tormenting. He only escaped the demeaning comments and physical assaults when he went off to a state college and from that point on, he left his parent's home for good.

John majored in elementary education and met a "hippy" young woman in one of his classes who taught him about meditation and invited him to a campus meditation group that she regularly attended. John became a regular at the group's weekly meetings where he would spend at least an hour a week sitting cross-legged on a zafu, engaging in various guided meditations. While focusing on images of tranquility and strength, or simply focusing on the inflow and outflow of his breath, John attained at least temporary respite from images of his own perceived inadequacy and feelings of self-doubt. He continued his meditative practice throughout college and now, as an elementary education teacher, continues to attend meditation groups and to practice daily.

According to John, the benefits of meditation evolved slowly, but the more he practiced, the more benefit he attained. At first the mindfulness practice served only to temporarily take his mind away from perceptions of worthlessness. The next stage was the development of an attitude of acceptance and a nonjudgmental stance toward others. He states that a big step for him was developing a nonjudgmental view of his parents whom he saw as emotionally limited and perhaps disturbed because of their own problematic and deficient upbringings. John often practices a loving-kindness meditation, and this has allowed him to be more accepting of himself and less self-judgmental. Next, he practiced acceptance and love toward all living beings, human and nonhuman.

John reports that his meditation practice, which he asserts will continue for the rest of his life, has resulted in a deep philosophical shift within him. He describes this shift as a movement toward seeing everyone as interconnected and deserving of kindness and love, including himself. John has been transformed from an insecure, self-critical, negativistic person into a loving and wise individual. Abuse-focused therapy has also helped John come to terms with his traumatic past and to develop an awareness of how this past has impacted him. John's romantic relationship has continued to blossom because of the gains brought about by his meditation and dealing with his own abuse history in therapy. John wishes to have children and states that he has every intention of making sure that he provides them the unconditional love and nurturance that he did not receive. He happily reports that he has asked the woman he is seeing to marry him, and she agreed. By his own account, John reports that dedicated meditation practice has been the basis of his major personal transformation.

## 10.14 Summary

Frontline workers, health service providers, family members, and others who have been negatively impacted by the trauma of others can find relief, fulfillment, and rejuvenation in the practice of meditation. Meditative practice has a long history and is often associated with specific religions, but in the West, it has lost much of its association with religion and is simply employed as a technique to promote well-being. Its popularity is attested to by the fact that computer searches show tens of thousands of applications for which mindfulness is said to provide benefits. The practice of mindfulness requires both commitment and sustained practice. It is not an easy skill to attain. One must commit to developing sustained attention to reduce the continued interference of intruding thoughts, and one must also give meditation priority so that it is practiced daily, often for a lifetime. Meditation can use specific images involving acceptance, love, tranquility, or strength or simply involve focused attention on breathing or body sensations. Empirical research supports the use of mindfulness practice for both the alleviation of emotional distress and the enhancement of feelings of fulfillment, tranquility, and regard for oneself and others. As such, meditation can be of significant benefit for those suffering the debilitating effects of secondary traumatization.

# Chapter 11
# Yoga and Secondary Trauma

It is reasonable to ask why a practice involving stretching, balance, and body positions might be of any value in managing psychological distress, whether it be from secondary trauma, primary trauma, or PTSD. In fact, yoga has been used for those purposes and others and has been practiced for approximately five thousand years. In Sanskrit, the term is translated as "union" or "connection." More than 16 million people practice yoga regularly (Emerson & Hopper, 2011) in the USA. The National Center for Complementary and Alternative Medicine (CAM) (2014) defines yoga as "A mind and body practice with origins in ancient Indian philosophy. The various styles of yoga typically combine physical postures, breathing techniques, and meditation or relaxation. There are numerous schools of yoga. Hatha yoga, the most practiced in the United States and Europe, emphasizes postures (*asanas*) and breathing exercises (pranayama). Some of the major styles of hatha yoga are Iyengar, Ashtanga, Vini, Kundalini, and Bikram yoga" (para. 1). Yoga facilitates awareness of a connection between physiological and mental states (Kaley-Isley et al., 2010) regardless of the age of the participants and can be effective in managing and dealing with traumatic experiences because of its ability to integrate somatic and mental/emotional states.

What one finds in those who are traumatized is that there is a separation between the body and mental/emotional states. The traumatized individual knowingly or unknowingly attempts to push away or separate themselves from the aversive experience of the trauma, regardless of the nature of that trauma (e.g., Motta, 2020). When one is engaged in yoga practice, there is a heightened awareness of the body, and the required attention given to body positions and stretches necessitates an integration or tying together of body and mental states. Yoga thereby counters the normal tendency among trauma victims to create distance from negative mental/emotional responses to trauma and facilitates a needed integration.

Van der Kolk (2014) advocates yoga for those suffering from trauma because the body is said to be the primary recipient or target of trauma, as the title of his popular book *The Body Keeps the Score* suggests. He offers different points of view as to the

© The Author(s), under exclusive license to Springer Nature Switzerland AG 2023

R. W. Motta, *Secondary Trauma*, https://doi.org/10.1007/978-3-031-44308-4_11

causes of yoga's effectiveness and speculates that when one maintains an effortful body position and then attains relief after the time has elapsed for holding that position, this might provide an expectation that other discomforts such as those due to trauma also have an end. Again, van der Kolk (2014) maintains that trauma is experienced primarily in the body and that yoga, with its focus on body positions and stretches (asanas), is therefore a reasonable way to deal with traumatic experiences. Yoga reportedly integrates emotional, cognitive, and physiological states. He further suggests that heart rate variability (HRV), a purported reflection of sympathetic and parasympathetic nervous system responses, is not synchronized with emotional states in those who are traumatized. For example, the traumatized individual might show excessive cardiac activity in response to ostensibly nonthreatening situations because those situations are interpreted as dangerous. Recordings of HRV in this case would show wave patterns that are out of sync with expected or normal HRV. By studying HRV one is provided with electrophysiological data that supplements verbal reports of the efficacy of yoga in managing traumatic experiences. With dedicated yoga practice, the HRV recordings of traumatized individuals begin to resemble those of people who have not been traumatized, suggesting that mental/emotional and physiological states have now become integrated.

Another neurophysiological explanation for the value of yoga is provided by Weintraub (2012, p. 14) who states, "On a biochemical and physiological level, previous research has shown that yoga relaxes chronic muscle tension, restores natural diaphragmatic breathing, improves oxygen absorption and carbon dioxide elimination, increases alpha and theta brain waves, and regulates the thalamus at an optimum level." Yoga is said to facilitate self-regulation (e.g., Dick et al., 2014), stress physiology (e.g., Riley & Park, 2015), and interoceptive awareness (van der Kolk, 2006).

Regardless of whether the data in support of yoga for dealing with trauma is verbal, electrophysiological, or biochemical, yoga is an empirically supported and widely popular way of coping with distress. Virtually every city and town in the USA has access to yoga instruction, and the Internet has made such access available to virtually everyone worldwide. Yoga has also found a home in most Veterans Health Administration Centers for the treatment of various kinds of traumas arising from a variety of military activities (Motta, 2020).

## 11.1 Mind-Body Interaction vs. Bodymind

Consider for a moment a therapist who spends multiple hours per day dealing with those who have been sexually assaulted. The therapist might develop secondary trauma symptoms owning to emotional depletion resulting from constantly supporting trauma victims. This therapist might also be plagued by images of violent assaults and the helplessness of victims. To cope with these emotional demands, the therapist attempts to distance themself from vicariously experienced, or secondary traumas, but not dealing with these traumas can result in their transfer into the body.

The result can be a variety of physiologically negative consequences, such as high blood pressure, digestion problems, and ulcers (e.g., van der Kolk, 2014). In this case mental or emotional states appear to have caused a negative reaction in the body, and this is the classic mind-body conceptualization of distress. It is a temporal or causal interpretation of how our minds cause havoc in our bodies. Psychological stress is seen as preceding and "causing" unhealthy body responses. By uniting body and mind, as is said to occur in yoga practice, one might be better able to forestall or avoid this negative causal sequence.

As was previously noted in Chap. 9 where exercise was shown to be of benefit for managing secondary traumatization, a "bodymind" model (Pert, 1999) was found to clarify the underlying mechanism for this benefit. Pert's view, based on her research on how neurochemicals and emotional states are intertwined (Pert et al., 1985), is that the notion of the two separate entities of mind and body having an impact on each other does not provide a precise picture of what is taking place. In her view, traumatic experiences impact body and mind not because of a hypothesized causal link or temporal sequence but rather because body and mind are one single entity (bodymind), not separate entities. In Pert's conceptualization, the mental/emotional and somatic consequences of trauma occur together, rather than taking place in a sequential manner. Neurochemical changes precipitated by stressful experiences are registered physiologically as well as mentally/emotionally because of the union of mental, emotional, and physiological processes. We interpret these neurochemical alterations as having a sequential effect, but the bodymind model implies no such temporal sequence. Bodymind implies a simultaneous alteration of mental/emotional and physiological states. Yoga practice emphasizes bodymind awareness through engagement in asanas.

Yoga facilitates our awareness of the integration of these states and combats the suppression or avoidance of experienced trauma. The notion that the body and mind are unitary has historical precedent. Pert has provided neurochemical evidence for views whose provenance dates to ancient Rome (mens sana in compore sano—a healthy mind in a healthy body) and more recently to Jacobson who claimed that an anxious mental/emotional state cannot exist when the body is relaxed (Jacobson, 1938), and that is where the value of yoga shows itself in the treatment of secondary traumatic states. Yoga can be said to provide health for the "bodymind." It is an integration practice.

## 11.2 Research Findings

The two functional processes that appear to become linked in the practice of yoga are mind and body states, or "bodymind" states (Pert, 1999). Researchers have found that increases in mindfulness, or being present, which is a key component of yoga, are associated with reductions in anxiety, depression, and PTSD (e.g., Bussing et al., 2012; Uebelacker et al., 2010). There are virtually no studies specifically designed to investigate the impact of yoga and secondary trauma per se, but one does find abundant research on components and correlates of secondary trauma such as anxiety, depression, and PTSD. Yoga focuses on physical activity, balance, and strength. Physical activity, in and of itself, is associated with reductions in anxiety, depression, and PTSD, as shown in Chap. 9. Van der Kolk (2014) suggests that yoga is capable of "rewiring" the brains of those who have experienced trauma of various kinds by specifically activating areas of the brain associated with trust, pleasure control, and social engagement and deactivating anxiety and depressive reactions.

There are not a huge number of randomized controlled studies or trials (RCTs) that are specifically oriented to investigating the effects of interventions such as yoga, but such studies do exist. In a meta-analysis performed by Gallegos et al. (2017), 19 RCT-type studies were included, and these were specifically oriented toward investigating the impact on trauma responses of various complementary therapies such as yoga and meditation. Overall findings were that these forms of intervention had a statistically significant impact on trauma and negative emotional states, but the effect sizes were small to medium. A value of such interventions is that they are readily available, do not require medically and psychologically trained professionals, and are not considered to be formal "therapies" and therefore less likely to be avoided by those who experience secondary traumatic stressors.

Studies that combine and summarize the findings of the impact of yoga on depression, which is a common characteristic among those who experience secondary trauma, have found statistically significant positive effects of yoga (e.g., Cramer et al., 2013; da Silva et al., 2009; Mehta & Sharma, 2010). These results are more impressive when it is realized that yoga was used as a standalone treatment and not as an adjunct to other therapies. Similar reviews show positive impacts of yoga on anxiety (e.g., Fortylow, 2011; Kirkwood et al., 2005; Li & Goldsmith, 2012).

In addition to studies relevant to yoga's impact on anxiety and depression, reviews have also found yoga to be a beneficial treatment for PTSD (da Silva et al., 2009; Fortylow, 2011; Longacre et al., 2012; Telles et al., 2012). Many of these studies included those who witnessed distressing events such as those who were diagnosed as having secondary trauma. Specific components identified as beneficial in yoga for trauma were breathwork, posture, and meditation (Longacre et al., 2012).

Macy et al. (2018) conducted a "meta-review" of 13 literature reviews on the impact of yoga on anxiety, depression, and PTSD. This review included 185 individual studies and found the impact of yoga on mental health to be "encouraging but preliminary" (p. 1). In general, the quality of the research was lacking in rigor with considerable differences in the methodologies, measures, and study samples. Nevertheless, these authors concluded that there was ample evidence for yoga, at least as an adjunctive treatment, for the treatment of a variety of negative affective states specifically seen in trauma-exposed individuals. It is well-known that individual studies in any area of inquiry should not be seen as definitive. What is impressive about the Macy et al. review of reviews of yoga is that it included numerous studies, and these supported the use of yoga for trauma and related disorders.

## 11.3 Yoga for the Traumatized

According to Harrison (2018), there are approximately 30 types of yoga that are practiced in the USA, but certain modifications of these practices should be considered when working with those who are traumatized. Traumatized individuals, whether they have experienced primary trauma as is seen in PTSD or are suffering from secondary trauma due to the nature of their work in which they are continually giving of themselves, often have difficulty with the many standard yoga practices. The reason this is so is that most yoga practices are directed and scripted and presented in such a way that direction and control are in the hands of the yoga instructor. Traumatized individuals often feel out of control of the daily situations they confront, and they find this lack of control of their environments to be aversive (Motta, 2020). For this reason, Emerson and Hopper (2011) advocate a form of yoga where the presentation allows for flexibility and choice. In such an approach, the traumatized yoga student can choose to alter the specifics of the asanas (postures), choose how long to hold a given asana, and choose not to be guided, directed, or physically touched by the instructor. This placement of choice in the hands of the trauma sufferer rather than those of the instructor is essential for traumatized individuals regardless of the form of the specific yoga practice.

## 11.4 Case Presentation

Jill's experience with trauma began at the tender age of 4. Her father's attentions at first seemed playful and loving. He would hug her, toss her playfully in the air, and cuddle with her. These displays of affection quickly progressed to touching and stroking Jill's genitals and then having her masturbate him. With time these encounters progressed into mutual oral sexual activity and then, by age 7, to intercourse. She was threatened with physical harm should she ever mention a word about what was taking place and was also informed that she would destroy the family if she said anything. Although she dreaded her father's attentions, she survived by not dealing with them and not letting them occupy her conscious thoughts. This process is a form of "dissociation" and is a way of dealing with extremely disturbing and anxiety-provoking situations. They are pushed from consciousness. Her sexual abuse continued until the age of 17 and would have continued beyond that had she not mentioned it to a friend in high school.

The friend reported the abuse to the school psychologist who contacted child protective services. Jill's father was arrested, jailed, and, in the process of preparing for trial, suffered a minor stroke. Jill's emotional distress over the abuse and its consequences to her family led to a suicide attempt involving the ingestion of a bottle of medication her mother had been taking to lower her blood pressure. Following a 3-week hospitalization, Jill entered an outpatient program of psychotherapy and received antidepressant medication. Jill was eventually able to come to terms with what happened to her although she continues to express bitterness and hate for her father. She eventually graduated from college where she majored in psychology because of her natural interest in that area of study and because of a need to better understand herself, especially her distrust in relationships. She has continued in therapy and with a low dose of antidepressants. In addition to emotional difficulties, Jill reports a long history of stomach pains and digestive problems but, despite having seen several physicians, has not been told of any specific medical problem that would explain her physical distress.

Just prior to graduating from college and continuing after college, Jill began volunteering as a hotline counselor. The work was challenging in that many of the calls she handled were from those who expressed the desire to kill themselves. Some of these calls were from people who had been involved in destructive relationships, those who had lost control of their addictions, and people like her who had been sexually abused. Jill felt some degree of satisfaction in being able to help others. She felt that her dismal childhood and adolescent experiences of abuse were being put to good use in that they allowed her to empathize with those who were in emotional distress, especially those who had experienced childhood sexual abuse. The downside of her hotline work was that she was becoming increasingly burdened and burnt out by what seemed to be an endless stream of phone calls of wrenching psychological pain. In Jill's particular case, her personal trauma history when combined with her hotline work provided a fertile environment for the development of secondary trauma and compassion fatigue. Her digestive issues became increasingly burdensome, and she started experiencing stomach cramping, which seemed to be at their worst on Sunday evenings when the new workweek loomed ahead. Jill tried an array of over-the-counter medications to alleviate her stomach and digestive distress, but these had little impact. A coworker told Jill about a yoga class that she was attending, and Jill decided to give it a try.

Things did not go well for Jill when she began her yoga classes. There was something about being directed to assume certain body positions and holding them that precipitated feelings of apprehension on Jill's part. After discussing her reactions with her therapist, she concluded that the format of the yoga sessions in which you are instructed to assume certain positions that were unnatural bore some similarity to being forced to engage in illicit sexual encounters by her father. At first Jill found this explanation to be farfetched, but upon reflection, it did seem a possible reason as to why directed body postures would be so unsettling for her. She decided to discuss her discomfort with the yoga instructor. The instructor reported that she had encountered similar reactions from other students and surmised that Jill might have experienced some form of physical trauma. This yoga instructor recommended another class to Jill where the instructor was skilled in working with those who have experienced trauma.

When applied by a skilled practitioner, yoga can have clear therapeutic effects. "This should be of no surprise when we realize that a common denominator of all traumas is a disconnection from the body and a reduced capacity to be present in the here and now" (Emerson & Hopper, 2011, p. xi). Jill began her new "trauma-focused yoga" group and almost immediately felt more at ease and far more able to complete the various postures (asanas) that were prescribed. But why, she wondered would this be the case? Both her former class and this one required the holding of certain difficult body positions for periods of time. When she asked the instructor, what the difference was between the classes, it was explained to her that there were several differences but two were especially important. First, the instructor was far less directive. For example, rather than say "extend your left arm forward and raise your right leg," this instruction would now be preceded by "if you feel comfortable, you may wish to try extending your left arm …" This alteration in instruction gave control over to the student, whereas previously, control resided with the instructor. The student was allowed to do things in their own way or not do it at all, and this was acceptable. Traditional yoga instruction is far more directive. A second important difference is that the yoga instructor never made physical contact with the student. In typical yoga teaching, the instructor will often physically assist the student to attain the correct posture by, for example, lifting a leg or putting their hands on the practitioner's shoulders. This physical touch and direction, especially in a person with Jill's sexual abuse history, set off immediate alarm sirens and an almost reflexive reaction to withdraw. In all, trauma-focused yoga gives control over to the student and is seldom directive, forceful, evaluative, or confrontive. Some forms of yoga are highly scripted and must be followed precisely, often requiring physical contact. This is the antithesis of trauma-focused yoga where there is no physical contact and far greater flexibility is allowed in attaining various body postures.

Despite initial apprehensions, Jill took well to her new trauma-focused yoga classes and, for reasons she could not articulate, felt a sense of peace and tranquility after her sessions. Within the first few sessions, she also began to experience a reduction in her stomach and digestive distress. She felt a renewed connection with her body (Emerson & Hopper, 2011) and no longer felt that it was an entity causing her distress. Yoga, in combination with Jill's ongoing psychotherapy and her low dose of antidepressant medication, allowed her to be better able to cope with and accept the stressors of her hotline work. The responding to desperate callers continued to be stressful for Jill, but the level of stress was now far more manageable. Jill now had an escape route. When the stress levels began to build and she began experiencing physiological distress, she would attend additional yoga classes, and this turned out to be tremendously beneficial to her. As so aptly stated by van der Kolk (2014) "the body keeps the score" as far as trauma is concerned. As a result, the body and mind-focused intervention of yoga can be surprisingly beneficial in alleviating that trauma, as it was in Jill's case of secondary trauma.

## 11.5 Specific Yoga Practices

Specific yoga practices differ in several ways including whether they are for beginners, intermediate, or advanced practitioners. They also differ in the precision required for completion of asanas; the rigidity of the sequence of asanas; the temperature of the space in which the practice takes place; the overall vigor or activity level of the practice; the degree to which meditation is part of the yoga practice; whether the meditation emphasizes focus (dharma), or absorption (dhyana), or oneness (samadhi); the degree to which specific breathing techniques are practiced (pranayama); and others. Twelve of the more popular forms of yoga (Harrison, 2018) include the following:

- *Anusara*: involves gentle exercise for people of various fitness levels, creates positivity and joy, and is good for strength and flexibility. This gentle approach might be suitable for those experiencing secondary trauma.
- *Ashtanga*: aimed at the most committed of students. The same asanas are practiced in the same order. It involves vigorous exercise and will help with overall fitness. The highly structured nature of this practice might not be received well by many trauma sufferers.
- *Bikram*: like Ashtanga, there is a specific sequence of asanas, but it is practiced in a heated room so that the body temperature rises, and this helps the muscles relax and become more flexible. The heat level can create dangerous core temperatures. It is not good for beginners and perhaps not for those experiencing secondary trauma.
- *Hatha*: one of the oldest and most popular forms of yoga that incorporates gentle physical activity, healthy diet and lifestyle changes, flexibility, and mental focus. The flexible nature of this technique might be suited for traumatized individuals.
- *Iyengar*: a very precise form of yoga that may use straps, blocks, chairs, and blankets to get the exact alignment of the body. It is slow and methodological and is seen as beneficial for physical injuries such as spinal disorders. Its directive nature and demands on precision may not make it ideal for the emotionally traumatized.
- *Jivamukti*: a lesser-known form of yoga emphasizing vigorous activity, spirituality, and meditation on nonviolence and non-harming and employing music.
- *Kripalu*: the gentlest form of yoga and is based on self-compassion. It is soft and slow, and its gentle focus on body awareness makes it suitable for the elderly and those who may not be in good physical condition. This form of yoga might be perceived as nonthreatening and non-anxiety-provoking for those who are traumatized and therefore would be of benefit to them.
- *Kundalini*: a highly spiritual form of yoga that includes challenging breath exercises (pranayama) coupled with asanas, mantra chanting, and meditation.
- *Sivananda*: like Hatha yoga but has more of a focus on breath and is one of the more spiritual forms. It also emphasizes diet (vegetarian) and positive thinking.
- *Viniyoga*: an advanced type of yoga that incorporates specific breathing exercises (pranayama) and long periods of asanas to increase inner focus, insight, and awareness. It is slow and calming.
- *Vinyasa*: one of the most energetic and popular forms of yoga where there is a focus on precise asanas and the transitions between them. Music is often played in sessions. Variation is allowed in the order of asanas, and it is an excellent exercise. The demands for precision might not sit well with those who have been impacted by trauma.

- *Yin*: focuses on meditation, flexibility, and exercise. The poses are held for a few minutes each, and this allows for the development of meditative skills and inner awareness. It is a great practice for beginners and can complement other forms of yoga. Given this description, it might be well received by traumatized participants.

## 11.6 Less Formalized Types of Yoga

Harrison (2018) also describes many other lesser-known and atypical forms of yoga. They are presented here to provide the reader with an appreciation of the extremely wide variety of yoga practices that have been promulgated. They are not necessarily considered to be serious approaches to treating those who have been traumatized. Some of these yoga practices involve "raves" and include the use of drugs. Yoga raves are said to be popular in Argentina, Uruguay, Paraguay, Chile, Brazil, Denmark, Sweden, Berlin, and the USA. Horse yoga involves doing yoga while riding a horse. Aerial yoga can involve practicing asanas dangling from ropes or from hammock-like supports. Karaoke yoga involves singing along with an electronic model while doing yoga. Yoga is done with pets such as cats, dogs, and other animals including farm animals. There is also a form of yoga called "cannabis yoga" that incorporates various methods of cannabis ingestion while engaged in yoga practice. Alcohol use versions of yoga also exist. There are many other types with names such as tantrum yoga, mommy-and-me yoga, paddleboard yoga, and others. These are included only to give the reader an idea of the wide-ranging popularity of yoga and the range of its variations. And while some of these later presented forms of yoga may come across as both frivolous and fanciful, yoga is nevertheless a serious health practice that can be of value in helping the traumatized escape from their trauma and help them integrate the physical and emotional aspects of their functioning.

## 11.7 Summary

Individuals experiencing secondary trauma and other forms of traumatization such as PTSD can benefit from the nontraditional therapeutic intervention of yoga. Yoga has been a source of stress alleviation that has been practiced for centuries. Yoga involves a combination of body postures (asanas), breathing techniques (pranayama), meditations, and sometimes includes healthy lifestyle and spiritual components. The commonly accepted view of why yoga is helpful in managing traumatic states is that it yokes body and mind states, which are seen as having been separated because of having experienced trauma. The "disintegration" of these states is "reintegrated" by engaging in a practice that requires a unification of body and mind. The concept of bodymind was presented as an alternative conception to the view that mental/emotional states impact physiological states. In the bodymind concept, there are no separate states of body and mind but rather a unitary state that is negatively impacted by trauma. Neurophysiological and electrophysiological data were presented supporting the importance of yoga for creating greater harmony between mental/emotional and physiological functioning.

Several research reviews were presented including randomized controlled trials (RCT) in support of yoga for dealing with trauma and the anxiety and depression that often accompany traumatic experiences. Twelve of the most common forms of yoga were described including those that may or not be advised for those suffering from trauma. Other atypical types of yoga were also presented to give the reader an appreciation of how widespread and varied yoga has become. In all, yoga is one of several potentially viable avenues and resources for those who suffer from secondary traumatization. It is not presented as a formal therapy for secondary trauma but rather as a way of promoting healthy functioning among those who have become emotionally debilitated by the nature of their work with those who are distressed.

# Chapter 12
# The Impact of Animals on Secondary Trauma

The human-animal interaction can be significantly beneficial in dealing with various forms of trauma including secondary traumatization. According to Hajar (2015), the presence of animals can reduce stress, anxiety, and depression and encourage exercise and playfulness while providing unconditional love and affection. Humans have kept animals as pets for the purpose of stress reduction and as companions throughout history. Archaeologists have uncovered the remains of a puppy cradled in the hands of a human from as early as 10,000 BCE. A cat was found buried with a human in Cyprus dating back to 7500 BCE. Ancient Egyptian paintings depict house cats around 3000 BCE and cats were sacred in ancient Egypt. Pets have been associated with health benefits including lowering blood pressure, and, in general, pet owners have lower levels of cardiac disease, heart failure, strokes, and other circulatory ailments (Abdill & Juppe, 2005; Hajar, 2015). There is a bond between animals and humans, and this bond has been found to ameliorate stress of both physical and psychological origin. The bond can have a downside. Studies show that veterinarians experience significant emotional distress that is akin to secondary trauma when their actions inadvertently cause harm to animals under their care (Kogan et al., 2018). This distress in response to harming an animal highlights the close bond that we have formed with animals.

Wompold (2015) reports on the outcomes of a series of meta-analyses that show the relationship and the ability to form this relationship which is the curative element in therapy, more so than are the therapeutic techniques or methods that are employed. Similarly, in the foreword of their book on the development of resilience that is fostered by relationships with animals (Tedeschi & Jenkins, 2019, p. xi), it is asserted that "a helping relationship is the best predictor of (therapeutic) outcomes independent of clinical technique or therapeutic perspective." Many animals, and particularly dogs, have a remarkable capability to form such relationships with humans. Dogs and humans appear to have had a codependent relationship that goes back 32 thousand years (Tedeschi & Jenkins).

© The Author(s), under exclusive license to Springer Nature Switzerland AG 2023

R. W. Motta, *Secondary Trauma*, https://doi.org/10.1007/978-3-031-44308-4_12

The essential benefit of relationships, whether human or animal, may be that they provide the comfort of not feeling alone and feeling less vulnerable. Aloneness is such an aversive experience that it is often used as the ultimate punishment as when one is placed in solitary confinement by corrections facilities. Humans are social animals, but nevertheless, they are animals and like many species of animals are evolutionarily programmed to seek social groups and relationships. When secondary trauma produces feelings of isolation and an urge to withdraw, contact with animals can diminish the feeling of being alone and can facilitate an inclination to seek social contact with others (e.g., Beetz et al., 2019; O'Haire & Rodriguez, 2018).

Abdill and Juppe (2005) describe the value of animals in health-care facilities. These facilities might be for the aged, emotionally troubled, intellectually challenged, or medical settings. These authors assert that "An animal's unconditional, unbiased, and abiding love is very rewarding to witness in action. It elicits smiles, encourages movement, and stimulates conversation, play and interaction. Love from an animal encourages reminiscing, provides nurturing, and produces enjoyment. It encourages therapeutic touch, increases self-esteem and, most importantly, provides a home-like atmosphere in any setting" (p. 7).

The use of animals to facilitate emotional growth was even noted by Sigmund Freud who included his dog, Jofi, in his therapy sessions. He claimed that the dog's unconditional acceptance of clients without regard to their anxieties and other emotional difficulties encouraged the clients to reveal and deal with their difficulties to a greater degree than if the dog was not present (Beck, 2010). Florence Nightingale (1969) remarked upon the value of animals in facilitating healing and accelerating positive outcomes in medical facilities. St. Elizabeth's Hospital in the early 1900s used animals for the purpose of facilitating recovery from various medical procedures (Huck & Burk, 2019). In 1980 researchers at the University of Pennsylvania reported that the presence of pets resulted in increased longevity among those who had suffered heart attacks (Abdill & Juppe, 2005). These findings are in accord with the observations of other researchers who report on the significant value of pets in facilitating both psychological and medical well-being (e.g., Eggiman, 2006; Parish-Plass, 2008; Rodriguez et al., 1996; Sobo et al., 2006).

In discussing the stress-reducing capabilities of animals, Tedeschi and Jenkins (2019) assert that animals often have superior senses such as olfaction, sight, and hearing and as a result can provide an alerting function of potential danger to humans. "When a dog is present and projecting nonverbal, nurturing signals, part of the human brain knows 'the camp is safe'" (Tedeschi & Jenkins, 2019, p. xii). Similarly, if the dog is playful and emotionally responsive, humans interpret their behavior as meaning that the environment, in general, is one in which they can feel secure. If the dog is startled and aroused, the message to humans might be one of vigilance and alertness being needed. People who are secondarily traumatized have been negatively impacted emotionally by others who are in distress. The presence of a calm, responsive, and emotionally connected animal provides assurance that there is little to be concerned about.

Another important therapeutic element that evolves from human interaction with animals is animals' ability to elicit emotionally regulated functioning. The process of petting, grooming, walking, riding, and simply attending to the activities of animals has a calming somatosensory effect. Surprisingly, these positive effects have also been found to be brought about even by plush (stuffed imitation) animals. Abdill and Juppe (2005) report a study in which residents in a long-term care facility who were provided with plush animals showed significant improvements in psychological well-being, social interaction, mental alertness, life satisfaction, and lower levels of depression in comparison to a control group who were not provided with stuffed animals. It was theorized that the beneficial impact of the plush animals was due to their representing real animals with whom the residents had prior beneficial reactions. Abdill et al. note that a wide array of animals has been shown to have a beneficial impact on human psychological functioning, including dogs, cats, horses, rabbits, llamas, pigs, hamsters, and many others. Even fish and reptiles that don't readily form bonds with humans can enhance one's sense of self-efficacy and self-confidence through effective management and caring for them.

## 12.1 Service Animals and Trauma Reactions

There are two contexts when considering the role that animals might play in ameliorating secondary traumatic stress such as compassion fatigue. The first is that of trained animals, most commonly dogs, that are specifically trained to assist those with trauma-related issues. These are often referred to as service dogs. The second is the presence of animals in general that are not trained but that are often considered to be an important member of a human family unit and with whom strong attachments are formed. This section will deal with service animals. There is a paucity of controlled research involving secondary traumatization and the role of animals, but there are a handful of well-controlled studies involving PTSD and service dogs. One such well-designed study is that of O'Haire and Rodriguez (2018).

In the O'Haire et al. study, military veterans with PTSD were paired with service dogs that were trained to promote a sense of safety and to deal with veterans who were having nightmares, panic reactions, depression, and withdrawal from the environment. Withdrawal is a common characteristic seen in various forms of psychological trauma regardless of whether the trauma is primary as in PTSD or secondary as in compassion fatigue. Traumatized individuals withdraw from the environment because it is the environment that is perceived as the source of distress. Withdrawal becomes a way of reducing the impact of aversive stimuli. In the O'Haire et al. study, a national sample of veterans who already had a service dog was compared to those who had applied for a service dog after having been honorably discharged from the military. There were 66 wait-list controls who had applied for a service dog and 75 who already had been assigned a Labrador retriever, golden retriever, and some mixed breeds. For those who had been assigned a service dog, they were required to attend an initial training period of 3 weeks where they lived in dormitories at the dog training site and where they engaged in structured activities with the dogs. The veterans helped in training the dogs to respond to specific commands, but the dogs were also trained to respond to situations in which the veteran may have been having a nightmare or a panic or anxiety attack or to provide a barrier between the veteran and oncoming people to whom the veteran might respond with apprehension. The dogs were even trained to remind veterans to take required medication. Except for having and not having a service dog and being involved in their training, all other factors were held constant between groups. If those in the group with dogs or those without dogs were receiving ancillary treatment for trauma, whether medical or psychological, they all continued to do so. The effort in this study was to keep things as naturalistic as possible to assure the generalization of findings to the "real world."

Overall findings of the O'Haire and Rodriguez (2018) study were that those with service dogs showed significantly lower scores on standardized measures of anxiety, depression, and PTSD in comparison to those without dogs. The former group also had more social interactions, fewer withdrawal and avoidance responses, less absentee issues from work, and fewer documented medical visits and medical interventions. In all, those with service dogs functioned far better psychologically, physiologically, and socially than those without service dogs.

There is no such thing as a perfect study, and this one is no exception. One could argue, for example, that all participants in this study were positively disposed to dogs because if they were not, they would not have voluntarily participated in the process of asking for a service dog in the first place. It is unclear what the findings would be for those who were not positivity-oriented toward dogs.

In another study Yarborough et al. (2018) conducted interviews with veterans who had service dogs. With few exceptions, veterans had highly favorable views of their dogs. In this study of 41 veterans and their dogs, it was found that the service dogs engaged in a series of specific behaviors that were found to be beneficial in ameliorating trauma effects. These behaviors included:

- Waking veterans from nightmares when the dog heard the veterans yelling and thrashing in the middle of the night.
- Nudging the veteran to orient them to the present when he or she was seen as entering a dissociative state.
- Enhancing emotional reactivity. The numbing and withdrawal typically seen in traumatized veterans are lessened by the demands of the dog for attention and affection.
- Enhancing physical activity. The dog's need for exercise and for feeding forces veterans to increase their level of activity and engage in behaviors such as shopping to ensure the well-being of their dog.
- Alerting. The dog might physically push on the veteran to alert them to the oncoming presence of strangers.
- Medication reduction. Overall, veterans with dogs require less medication for blood pressure, cholesterol control, and lower dosages of antianxiety and antidepressant medications.

Yarborough et al. (2018, p. 123) pointed out that despite the overall benefits, there are "a few substantial challenges to using service dogs as therapeutic agents ..."

People with service dogs may be seen by some as having a disability or in some ways come across as different, but the overall benefits were substantial in terms of the general functioning of those who had been traumatized. Also, there are people who don't react well to the presence of dogs. For example, there are those who are allergic to dogs and those who are fearful in the presence of even the smallest and least intimidating of dogs.

Curley et al. (2021) conducted a study involving 140 first responders, for example, police, firefighters, and paramedics. The purpose of the study was to determine how first responders reacted to the presence of service dogs. The researchers asserted that there is little research on the impact of nontraditional interventions that are aimed at ameliorating the negative impact on the psychological functioning of first responders. Some evidence was cited from a prior study that showed that the presence of canines within stressful environments allowed first responders to work more efficiently on activities that were crucial to completing their tasks (Foreman et al., 2017). Police officers who work in a K-9 unit often see the dog that is assigned to their unit as a friend, protector, and buffer from stress (Hart et al., 2000; Ives, 2016).

Curley et al. (2021) did not find statistically significant variations in psychological adjustment or help-seeking attitudes when comparing organizations with or without support dogs in the workplace. They attributed this lack of difference to the fact that there was little psychological maladjustment overall at the inception of the study. However, there were benefits observed in the qualitative comments of those working with support canines. Specifically, it was noted that the presence of support canines acted as a positive distractor and stress reliever among those who had positive attitudes toward dogs. Those who did not have positive attitudes, that is, those who saw dogs as messy and potentially disruptive, did not perceive any potential benefit. The authors of the study suggest that the findings show an overall beneficial impact of the presence of canines and suggest that the perceptions of those who are not fond of dogs should be considered when organizations are deliberating over supplementing their units with canines.

Studies involving the potential beneficial presence of dogs in alleviating psychological distress are often conducted with veteran groups as these studies are likely to have access to samples with clear symptoms of psychological distress such as PTSD. Onc such study was conducted by Beetz et al. (2019). In this study 29 soldiers were provided with psychotherapy plus the presence of a service dog (the experimental group). The control group was comprised of 31 soldiers who received psychotherapy only. The experimental group received four weekly sessions of 3 h each. During these sessions the soldiers engaged in grooming activities, play, and walks with the dogs. The dogs were accompanied by military dog handlers, and the dogs were specifically trained to work with those who had experienced trauma. The only difference between the experimental and control groups was the presence of dogs and their handlers in the experimental group, and both groups received psychotherapy provided by the veteran's health service administration. Data were collected at the beginning of the study, at the end, and at a 1-month and 3-month follow-up. Results showed a worsening of perspectives and values related to work and social adjustment in the control group and a statistically significant trend toward better values and increased social engagement in the experimental group with the dogs. These differences were maintained in the follow-up assessments. The mental wellness of the experimental group improved over the 4-week course of the intervention, particularly in the ability to experience joy. There was no clear trend showing a perceived reduction of stress in the experimental group compared to the control group, but the former group showed improved social interactions especially with the dog handlers. This is an important finding as there is a characteristic tendency of those with PTSD to evidence withdrawal from social activities. The authors point out that their findings are compelling in that the intervention was carried out for only four sessions. It was suggested that a more extensive intervention with dogs would likely have shown even more compelling data on the benefits of dogs as a supplement to standard psychotherapeutic intervention.

## 12.2 Pets, Trauma, and Stress-Related Problems

Regarding the influence of non-service trained animals on well-being, Schwarzmueller-Erber et al. (2021) compared the physical, social, and psychological well-being of horseback riders, dog owners, and non-pet-owning controls to determine if there were any differences among the groups. Pet attachment scores were found to be equivalent between the two animal-involved groups. Physical activity levels did not differ between dog owners and horseback riders, but both groups were more active than controls. Gender differences were found in that females showed greater attachment scores to their horses than did males. In both groups involving animals, psychological well-being was found to be correlated with the level of attachment to the animal whether it was a dog or horse. Psychological, physical, and social well-being did not differ between dog owners and horseback riders, but both groups scored significantly better than did the controls.

The Schwarzmuller-Erber et al. (2021) study is relevant to those who experience secondary traumatization and primary trauma such as PTSD. Traumatized people have a pronounced tendency toward social avoidance (Motta, 2020), and the Schwarzmuller et al. study revealed an increased level of social integration and well-being among those who are involved with animals when compared to those who do not have pets. The animals in that study were not trained therapy animals but simply pets. This beneficial impact of pets on interpersonal functioning has also been reported by other researchers (e.g., Smolkovic, 2012). In general, the findings reveal that those who can form attachments to animals also show improved social interaction skills. It might be that this connection involving animal attachment and social interaction is correlational rather than causal, but the above-noted studies (Beetz et al., 2019; O'Haire & Rodriguez, 2018) on the impact of therapy dogs for those with PTSD suggest a possible causal connection. The ability to form relationships with animals appears to generalize to the formation of human social relationships. It is almost as if being able to bond with an animal serves as a catalyst or facilitator for forming human interactions.

Horses are not usually trained to be service animals as are dogs. Nevertheless, they have been shown to benefit those who have stress-related disorders, such as secondary trauma. Lanning et al. (2018) conducted a study with veterans who had suffered from PTSD for decades. In this study 89 veterans were randomly assigned to an 8-week therapeutic horseback-riding group (THR) or to a control group. In the THR group, each of the eight sessions was 90 min. During the sessions the veterans first shared a meal with each other and then engaged with the horses in riding, grooming, and exercise activities. Rather than rely only on paper-and-pencil measures and self-reports, the investigator also recruited family members to report on the participants' functioning throughout the study. Overall results showed that there were clinically significant reductions in PTSD and depression in those in the THR group but not in the non-THR control group. While the authors were unable to present unassailable proof that the beneficial impact of engagement with horses is what led to the clinically significant improvements, this study does agree with others showing a beneficial impact of human-animal interaction.

Another study involving horses and traumatized veterans was conducted by Johnson et al. (2018), and their focus was on whether engagement with horses would result in increases in perceived coping self-efficacy, emotional regulation, and decreases in PTSD, loneliness, and isolation. Again, it is common for those who have been traumatized, whether the trauma is secondary or primary as in PTSD, to show elevations in loneliness and social isolation. In this study 29 soldiers with PTSD were randomly assigned to a therapeutic horseback-riding group (THR) and to a control group. Significant reductions in PTSD were found after 3 weeks with even greater reductions shown after 6 weeks. The areas of loneliness, social isolation, and emotional regulation were not shown to differ significantly between the THR and control groups. It is possible that if the study were extended beyond six sessions, significant reductions might have been shown. However, the fact that significant reductions were shown in levels of PTSD for those in the THR group attests to the beneficial impact that being associated with animals can have on those who have encountered, and been impacted by, trauma.

The importance of social support for ameliorating the impact of secondary traumatization was addressed in a prior chapter of this book. The advent of the COVID-19 virus and the need for quarantining has made this resource less available than it had previously been according to Nieforth and O'Haire (2020). Pets have been able to serve the role of ameliorating the stress of social isolation not only in secondary trauma and primary trauma but also within the general population experiencing the negative impact of COVID-19. The isolation brought about by attempts to limit exposure to COVID-19 is likely to produce trauma reactions (Liu et al., 2020) and overall distress. The beneficial role of pets, according to Nieforth and O'Haire, is multifaceted. Pets can provide a sense of constancy and predictability, and these tend to run counter to and lessen the impact of COVID-19 unpredictability and uncertainty. Pets also show unconditional positive regard and acceptance. They provide a haven from distressing news about what is happening in the general population. Pets also provide contact comfort at a time when contact with the physical environment and with people may produce some degree of unease and wariness. The bonds created between animals and humans can have a healing impact in the same way that human relationships facilitate healthy adjustment following traumatic experiences (e.g., Lopez-Zeron & Blow, 2017). "Initial evidence suggests that the emotional bond shared between people and animals may offer a source of nonjudgmental support as well as a source of positive regard.... Which may be important when human-to human bonds are not accessible" (Nieforth & O'Haire, 2020, p. S245). The available research appears to show that the interactions found between animals and humans are not only perceived as being pleasurable but also serve to reduce the probability of developing trauma reactions in response to the types of stressors seen in secondary trauma and PTSD (e.g., O'Haire et al., 2015).

When one is evaluating the data that supports or does not support the benefits of animals in cases involving distress and various forms of trauma, most of the studies rely upon self-report. Self-report can take the form of responses to questionnaires or responses on paper-and-pencil measures that have shown their psychometric value in terms of strong validity and reliability. One of the few exceptions was the Lanning (2018) study in which the reports of family members were used to supplement the responses of those who had been traumatized and who had participated in a horseback-riding intervention. However, this study too relied upon the subjective observations and opinions of family members. One of the few exceptions to studies that evaluated the impact of animals on those who have been traumatized and that did not primarily rely on self-report was a study by Pendry et al. (2014) involving troubled youngsters.

Pendry et al. (2014) randomly assigned youngsters to either a horseback riding or control group and measured cortisol levels of both groups on a pre-post intervention basis. The participants had been referred by school personnel and counselors because of emotional and behavioral difficulties arising from troubled backgrounds and children from the community to either a horseback-riding condition or a control condition that did not involve horses. The researchers collected six samples of cortisol at pre-intervention and a similar sampling at post-intervention. Lower cortisol levels are associated with stress reduction and lower levels of psychopathology (e.g., Lupien et al., 2009).

The activities that were associated with horses included grooming, walking, riding, feeding, and observing the interactions of horses with handlers. Cortisol samples were taken at various times during the day for both the horseback-riding group and the control group. Overall results revealed significant reductions in cortisol levels of those youngsters who were engaged with animals. The results of this study add to the wide range of controlled studies and anecdotal observations regarding the benefit of interacting with animals and add a layer of validity to the positive findings by using a measure that does not rely upon subjective reports. One might be able to argue that it was not simply the interaction with animals that resulted in the lower cortisol level, but that involvement with people was also taking place within this study. After all, those youngsters involved with animals had to have the assistance, guidance, and instruction of experienced adults to show them what to do with the horses, and this supportive interaction with adults could also have had a beneficial psychological impact. These sorts of critiques are difficult to address experimentally. Nevertheless, the reduction in cortisol levels in this group of troubled participants after interacting with horses and their handlers is entirely congruent with other studies and observations regarding the stress-ameliorating role of animals. The utility of animals in reducing trauma reactions, such as those eventuating from situations where individuals are called upon to give of themselves to the point of distress, appears to have abundant empirical and subjective observational support.

## 12.3 The Case of Ingrid Tubor, MD

Ingrid Tubor is a 56-year-old internist who works at a Veterans Health Administration (VHA) facility in Long Island, New York. Her primary clientele are veterans who served in the Middle East wars, the Vietnam War, and a few from the Korean War. Many of her patients have health-compromising habits of smoking, excessive drinking, lack of exercise, and unhealthy diets. Several of them appear to be addicted to opiate-based painkillers, some of which she has prescribed and some of which come from other sources including illegal ones. Over the years she has come to know many of her patients as regulars and knows their military and post-military histories well. She has formed a close relationship with them and has listened to their family and financial woes and often felt burdened by these stories. There are times when she feels a pang of guilt for her fortune of having a secure and well-paying job, medical benefits, and comparatively good health overall. She is often troubled by the fact that she provides medical advice that is often ignored. For example, she has several patients whose obesity, smoking, drinking, inactivity, and reluctance to take prescribed medications have led to heart attacks, diabetes, and emphysema. She has attended the funeral services of several elderly Vietnam-era veterans, who would probably have had several more years of life had they followed her medical advice.

Most evenings Dr. Tubor goes home in a state of emotional exhaustion. She has come to terms with the fact that compassion fatigue is part of her job. She will often have dinner with her husband who works as a certified public accountant for a nearby firm. She and her husband have been married for 25 years, and neither of them has been eager to have children. They have a loving relationship, but her husband has grown increasingly impatient over the years listening to a litany of medical problems of Dr. Tubor's patients, and as a result she often keeps these troubling issues to herself. This inability to share with her husband has led to some degree of distance between them. They continue to care for each other, but her husband's impatience has lessened the degree of emotional support she once felt in their marriage. The couple does have two dogs, however, and they provide a surprisingly good amount of comfort to Dr. Tubor. One of them, Ginger, is a golden retriever, and the other, Molly, is a standard poodle.

On a typical day, Dr. Tubor will come home with her thoughts swirling with the specifics of some medical problem encountered by one or more of her patients. She would love to come home and say to her husband, "I told Ron a million times to take his Lipitor, but he just would not listen. Now he is in the hospital with a second heart attack." This is what she would want to say, but she knows that her husband will not only be unresponsive but that his subsequent emotional detachment will ruin the evening for her as she ruminates over the fact that he is no longer as supportive as he used to be. As a result, she says nothing. Her solace comes from Ginger and Molly whose bounding and enthusiastic response to her arrival home distracts her from the burdens of her job. Sometimes Dr. Tubor talks to her dogs and describes her daily frustrations to them. Regardless of what she says, they are unconditionally accepting, loving, playful, and more than eager to spend time with her regardless of what she is saying. All these responses contrast with those of her husband who, though loving, is not responsive to her woes. Molly, in particular, seems to connect on a deep level with Dr. Tubor.

Dr. Tubor acquired Molly from a "puppy mill" that had rented out space in a local shopping mall. Of all the dogs she saw, Molly seemed the most alert and responsive to her. The salesperson claimed to have a poodle just like Molly and that poodles were one of the most intelligent of dogs. She remembers him saying, "Sometimes they (poodles) will look at you in the eye, and you get a weird feeling that they are almost human." He stated that most other dogs don't have the poodles' attention span and that poodles are generally healthy dogs. At the time Dr. Tubor thought these comments from the salesperson were simply hype, but she was nevertheless attracted to Molly's engaging response to her. Since then, she has learned that the seller was right. Molly seemed hyperalert to her moods and at times seemed to know when Dr. Tubor required additional affection and would lick her endlessly.

Perhaps no single event distressed Dr. Tubor more than the devastating consequences of the COVID-19 pandemic. Her typically stressful job became almost intolerable when several of her patients were hospitalized, became pulmonary invalids ever dependent on breathing assistance, or simply died at home or in the hospital. She had been treating some of these patients for many years and was familiar with their families, their medical histories, and their health-compromising habits. She had known some for more than two decades and was devastated to hear of their sudden death at home or after surviving for months on hospital ventilators.

The VA hospital where she worked, recognizing the stress on their personnel brought about by COVID-19, offered several support services. These included supportive "rap" groups and mindfulness meditation groups, and, recognizing the psychological benefits of exercise, the hospital hired a fitness trainer to work with them. Dr. Tubor took part in the meditation and rap groups. She recognized that complaints to her husband about the devastating impact of COVID would only result in his becoming even more remote.

According to Dr. Tubor, the rap and meditation groups helped while she was at the VA, but on coming home she would find herself ruminating about her patients and their ill-health. Ginger and especially Molly became the balm that helped to salve her emotional wounds. No matter how despondent she was on returning home, her "kids" would greet her with bounding enthusiasm and excitement. They communicated both love and connection to her and their needs to be fed, walked, and occasionally groomed were a major and pleasing distraction for Dr. Tubor. Molly almost seemed to understand the stress level that Dr. Tubor was experiencing and was able to provide the support that her husband was not willing to provide. According to Nieforth and O'Haire (2020), people turn to pets for emotional support in times of stress and particularly in times when human support is unavailable as was the case with Dr. Tubor's husband. These authors also report that during times of unpredictability, as has been the case during the COVID-19 pandemic, pets counter the anxiety arising from this unpredictability by always being there in a dependable and predictable manner. Regardless of whether Dr. Tubor was particularly stressed or not, Molly and Ginger would be there for her and present themselves as a constant in a world that seemed filled with uncertainty.

With the passage of time, the devastating impact of the COVID-19 pandemic began to abate, and as a result the number of medical crises that Dr. Tubor had to deal with lessened. The reduction in deaths and hospitalizations reduced Dr. Tubor's distress, and she felt less alienated from her seemingly detached husband. But, regardless of whether she was stressed or not, Molly and Ginger were always there for her. They were a constant in the life of a medical practice that brought about a good deal of unpredictability. Dr. Tubor once remarked that Ginger and particularly Molly may have saved her marriage. She states that her husband is a good man and that they love each other, but his inability to help shoulder the compassion stressors that she regularly experienced may have led to the collapse of her marriage if it were not for her loving, predictable, and supportive "canine kids." Dr. Tubor remarks that the salesperson was correct when he asserted that poodles and other intelligent breeds give an almost eerie sense of connectedness with humans. Molly will often stare into Dr. Tubor's eyes almost as if trying to read what stresses she is undergoing. All in all, Molly and Ginger have made Dr. Tubor's life richer and simply more fun than if they were not there for her.

## 12.4 Summary

Anecdotal reports, clinical observations, and empirically based control group studies converge upon attesting to the value of animals in alleviating the type of distress seen in secondary traumatization. The beneficial relationships between animals and human dates to at least 10,000 BCE and history reveal that cats were once revered in ancient Egypt. Meta-analytic studies attest to the crucial role of relationships in alleviating emotional distress, isolation, and alienation. And it is in this area of relationship formation that the presence of animals plays a key role in helping humans cope with distress. As a result, animals have been incorporated into psychotherapy sessions and even into medical facilities where their presence is associated with the facilitation of healing. Sigmund Freud is reported to have engaged his chow, Jofi, as an aide in his psychoanalytic sessions. Florence Nightingale advocated for the use of animals in hospitals because their presence accelerated healing processes. It appears that the unconditionally stable, positive relationship between animals and humans and the animals' lack of an agenda, other than seeking out and appreciating human contact, serve to promote healthy psychological growth in humans.

Much of the empirical work for investigating the role of animals in human functioning comes from studies with what are called service animals. These highly trained animals, usually dogs, are often employed in studies examining their roles with veterans suffering from PTSD. Overall findings are that the presence of service dogs results in significant reductions in veterans' PTSD, anxiety, and depression while enhancing activity level and social engagement. The latter is of critical importance as a common characteristic of those who are traumatized is a tendency toward social isolation. Social isolation is likely due to avoidance of an environment and people that have been previously seen as distressing. Work has also been conducted with first responders and service dogs. First responders often suffer from secondary traumatization, which results from exposure to the trauma of others. Overall findings are that service dogs have been a welcome addition to first responder organizations and serve the role of buffering personnel from emotional distress.

A large variety of animals that are not considered to be service animals has also been found to have a stress-buffering effect. One of the more common animals that have been studied is horses. The presence of horses has been found to increase social interaction and social skills and to reduce anxiety and depression. These studies have been conducted with both veteran and civilian groups. One compelling study moved beyond measurement by self-report and measured cortisol levels in emotionally troubled adolescents. This control group study found significant reductions in cortisol levels in addition to improved socialization skills following interaction with horses. Troubled youngsters who did not interact with horses did not show these benefits or reductions in cortisol.

Not everyone who is distressed will benefit from the presence of animals. There are those who consider certain animals as messy and as stimulating allergic reactions, or they might fear that being seen with a service animal may make them appear to have a weakness or disability. Overall, however, animals do appear to both soothe, elevate mood, and facilitate social interaction. One study on plush or imitation animals found a beneficial impact on residents in eldercare facilities and other health facilities. This helpful impact of the presence of inanimate objects may be due to the plush animals being seen as close to the real thing and thereby evoking positive responses on the part of residents. Animals that don't seem to readily bond such as reptiles or fish have also been shown to produce emotional benefits, perhaps because of the need to care for them.

Finally, a case was presented in which the developing compassion fatigue of a health-care professional was lessened by the presence of pets. What this case and the long history of observations and research show is that animals and humans often bond with and provide comfort for each other. This bond not only ameliorates distress but also provides joy, promotes an increase in activity, provides a sense of constancy and predictability, and activates beneficial physical contact. Overall findings from both observations and empirical studies provide convincing evidence of the value of animals in lessening the deleterious effects of secondary traumatization. For this reason, animals should be considered as one of several possible resources for alleviating negative emotional states especially those that are related to traumatic experiences including secondary trauma.

# Chapter 13
# Self-Care and Natural Environments

The position that has been taken in this book is that secondary trauma is usually not the sort of psychological distress that requires formal psychotherapy. If intervention is needed, often brief paraprofessional intervention is sufficient. There are certainly exceptions to this especially in situations where the indirect traumatic or secondary traumatic experience is so frightening or emotionally disruptive that the line separating secondary or vicarious trauma and PTSD becomes blurred. One can imagine, for example, that untrained workers at a passenger aircraft crash site whose job is to recover bodies and body parts might become so emotionally distressed that they meet all the *DSM-5* criteria of PTSD and require formal psychotherapy. In general, however, personnel such as first responders and health-care workers have been trained to emotionally manage the crises they routinely experience. They will sometimes experience emotional exhaustion and stress that falls within the domain of what is identified as secondary trauma. The same might be said of family members who take care of an ailing relative. Their compassion fatigue is just that. They are exhausted by the caring they provide, but their difficulties do not fall within the boundaries of what defines PTSD, and therefore they do not require psychotherapy per se. First responders, health-care workers and those assisting family members may benefit from brief, sometimes single-session interventions provided by paraprofessionals or minimally trained health personnel.

The range of situations that can produce secondary trauma is both wide and diverse. The spouses of first responders such as police officers may develop secondary trauma (Dwyer, 2005), as might investigators who examine the abuse of children through the Internet (Tehrani, 2016), and even teachers who serve in the role of supporting students who have been traumatized might themselves develop secondary trauma (Hydon et al., 2015). Family members of war veterans (Suozzi & Motta, 2004; Waysman et al., 1993), family members of those with serious medical illness (Boyer et al., 2002; Libov et al., 2002; Lombardo, 2007), first responders (Gilbert-Eliot, 2020), foster care providers (Hannah & Woolgar, 2018), and many other groups might benefit from some form of intervention that is not formal

© The Author(s), under exclusive license to Springer Nature Switzerland AG 2023

R. W. Motta, *Secondary Trauma*, https://doi.org/10.1007/978-3-031-44308-4_13

psychotherapy but may rather be a brief form of counseling or information provision. These less intense forms of assistance can often be offered by paraprofessional counselors or hotline workers who have received some amount of training but who do not have professional degrees such as seen among psychologists, psychiatrists, and social workers. Often the secondarily traumatized person simply wants someone to share their experience with and has little need for extensive psychotherapeutic intervention. Some of the many paraprofessional interventions for secondary trauma are addressed below. Also presented below are interventions that are self-initiated and do not involve others.

## 13.1 Debriefing of Trauma Experiences

A popular form of nonprofessional or paraprofessional intervention that was previously touched on in an earlier chapter is the controversial process of critical incident stress debriefing (CISD) (Mitchell, 1983). The CISD process involves a detailed retelling of the specifics of the traumatic encounter along with a description of the personal feelings and sensations that were involved. This process is expected to take place within 48–72 h of the traumatic event or events. The rationale for revisiting traumatic experiences soon after they occur is that it is important to deal with and process the trauma before it becomes embedded as occurs in cases of PTSD. CISD is controversial in that it may not be advisable to have people reconfront traumatic memories so soon after the event because this process can further disturb them at a time when they are just coming to terms with what happened and are most vulnerable (Phipps & Byrne, 2003). People may require time to process traumatic experiences so that these experiences lose some of the emotional disruptiveness that they initially had. Only after one has had time to process their trauma might they beneficially recall it and their feelings in response to the trauma. Their feelings might be too raw and upsetting to relate within 48–72 h, and doing so might cause an exacerbation of emotional upset.

Many first responder organizations have used a single-session CISD format (Deahl, 2000) even though it was not initially intended as a single-session process (Mitchell & Everly, 1997). One common form of traumatic experience that first responders deal with is vehicular accidents. CISD has been used for both those who are called in during the aftermath of an accident and with the accident victims themselves. Mayou et al. (2000) examined the use of CISD with a group of individuals traumatized by such accidents using a one-session format. In a 3-year follow-up, it was found that the group who had received this treatment showed increased travel anxiety, physical problems, and an overall decrease in psychosocial well-being in comparison to those who did not receive the CISD intervention. Phipps and Byrne (2003) suggest that "the effectiveness of CISD may be affected by the individual's present level of functioning, and trauma history" (p. 141). Those who have significant psychological impairment after a traumatic event and/or those who have a significant trauma history may not respond well to CISD. But, regardless of trauma history and level of psychological impairment, the Mayou study suggests that the brief CISD intervention done so soon after the vehicular accidents resulted in an exacerbation of negative outcomes.

Bryant (2021) reports on a British study in which burn victims were either assessed for trauma or assessed and then treated with a debriefing procedure within 2–19 days of their burns. Even though there were no differences in assessed baseline levels between the two groups, a follow-up 13 months later showed that those who had the debriefing had significantly elevated scores on PTSD, anxiety, and depression in comparison to those who had not been debriefed. Pitman (1989) contends that trauma memories are consolidated in the immediate aftermath of a trauma. If these memories are reactivated through a debriefing procedure, which takes place at a time of stress associated with the recency of the trauma, the memories become even more consolidated (Bos et al., 2014). In a sense the trauma memories become more embedded and resistant to being neutralized by the very debriefing procedure that was intended to reduce them.

Again, the problem with using CISD is that the intervention process, given its short duration, may activate and exacerbate trauma symptoms. By repeatedly going over the characteristics surrounding the event and the feelings associated with it, one is engaging in a process akin to prolonged exposure (PE) (Foa et al., 2007). PE can be helpful in reducing the emotional impact of trauma, but it is also known to produce high levels of anxiety and avoidance (Motta, 2020). The brevity of CISD with its exposure focus often does not permit the important following up on anxiety and avoidance responses that may have been elicited during the intervention. Follow-up is an important part of mental health interventions. Also, the fact that CISD is often rendered by paraprofessionals lessens the chances of effectively managing iatrogenic outcomes that may eventuate from the procedure itself.

Given the controversial nature of CISD, a variant of it was developed and referred to as critical incident stress management (CISM) (Mitchell & Everly, 1997). The essential differences between these two interventions are that the latter adds a component of learning how to manage anxiety, which in this case is referred to as stress inoculation training (SIT) (Michenbaum, 1985). In addition to the inclusion of SIT, CISM also involves a follow-up process rather than simply having a one-shot intervention. CISM is seen as an integrated system that incorporates pre-incident training, post-incident defusing, and, if needed, provision of further counseling and follow-up.

Richards (2009) compared CISD with CISM in a prospective study involving financial services personnel who had lived through bank robberies. The samples consisted of 225 individuals who took part in CISD and 229 who were involved with CISM. The CISD group took place within the branch environment and was initiated within 72 h of the attempted robberies. Sessions lasted 1.5–2 h. The CISD intervention involved discussion of participants' memories of the facts of what happened along with detailed discussion of their thoughts and emotions. In the CISM group, pre-robbery training was given on how to manage anxiety in response to trauma exposure. Interventions such as breathing training, progressive muscle relaxation, and workbook exercises containing information on how to cope with robberies were also involved. Participants of both groups completed standardized trauma measures 3 days post-robbery, and at 3-, 6-, and 12-month follow-ups. Results of the study were complex, and there were differences between CISD and CISM at various follow-up points, but overall findings were that "employees in the CISM group were less traumatized at later follow-up and the proportion of clinically significant cases was less than half the number in the CISD group" (p. 358). The fact that CISD and especially CISM can be carried out by those who are not professionally trained mental health practitioners increases the availability and utility of such procedures. Neither CISD nor CISM is a psychotherapy per se, but rather they are practical approaches that can be used to lessen the impact of traumatic experiences including those involved in secondary traumatization. In general, empirical findings support the CISM as a more comprehensive and effective approach than CISD in dealing with a variety of traumatic experiences.

## 13.2 Self-Management Procedures

In addition to the procedures that can be taught by paraprofessionals to help in managing secondary trauma, there are also several self-management methods that can be effective tools for ameliorating distress. This section will touch on only a few of them to give the reader some idea of what is meant by "self-management." The above section notes that CISM incorporates a stress inoculation training component (SIT) (Michenbaum, 1985), which is a set of procedures designed to manage one's anxieties. Anxiety reduction is critical in managing the distress of secondary trauma. Many of the components of SIT can be used in a self-management context.

In general, the most employed method of reducing anxiety is simply to avoid thoughts, images, sensations, memories, perceptions, and experiences that are reminders of anxiety-provoking events such as traumatic and/or secondarily traumatic experiences (Motta, 2020). By avoiding the anxiety-provoking stimuli, whether it is a thought, image, or so forth, anxiety elevations are also avoided. However, while avoidance works in reducing anxiety in the short run, the problem with avoidance is that one does not overcome the anxiety-provoking trauma as one simply does not deal with it. The way one becomes strengthened and better able to cope with present and future disturbances due to traumas is to learn strategies and techniques for coping with them.

One such strategy, stress inoculation training (SIT) (Michenbaum, 1985), involves an amalgam of techniques including *diaphragmatic* or *deep breathing* (Hooper et al., 2018). This form of breathing involves a deep, slow inhalation usually of 10 s and an equally slow exhalation of the same duration. The process can be repeated up to ten times perhaps three times per day. Training in diaphragmatic breathing is associated with reductions in anxiety and greater control over the fight-or-flight response in that one now possesses a tool for coping with anxiety-provoking situations. Diaphragmatic breathing is also said to result in improved vagal activity, which is associated with reduced blood pressure, reduced pulse rate, and reduced sympathetic nervous system activity (Hooper et al.). According to Sultanoff (2001), this form of breathing is what we once engaged in as infants before the development of adult anxiety, depression, and so on, which negatively affected the flow of air into our lungs. This author claims that breathing training is essentially training in remembering how we breathed at an early point in our lives before being impacted by the stressors of life.

*Cognitive restructuring* is another component of SIT and involves learning how to make alternative interpretations of the traumatic incidents that have occurred and how one's own thoughts might contribute to the distressing nature of the trauma. So rather than take the position that a particular event is intolerable and horrible in the extreme, one might train themselves to view traumatic events as unfortunate, hurtful, and distressing but not beyond the realm of normal occurrences. Similarly, rather than construing one's own responses as unbearably painful and impossible to deal with, to see them as normal responses to abnormal circumstances. Emotions that might be seen as being beyond tolerable are alternatively seen as unwelcome, unpleasant, and unwanted but not being the realm of tolerability (Ehlers & Clark, 2000; Ellis, 1975). This "restructuring" of one's cognitions not only lessens the emotional distress brought on by traumatic experiences but also facilitates the dealing with, rather than the avoidance of, these experiences. Avoidance as stated earlier is the primary way in which people deal with distressing events, and while effective in the short run, it in no way helps the sufferer deal with and overcome the negative effects of trauma.

*Thought stopping* is another self-control procedure that is associated with stress inoculation training (SIT). Thought stopping involves making a conscious effort to block the constant flow of negative and anxiety-producing thoughts. When these thoughts arise, an attempt is made to replace them with more positive and balanced alternatives. This can be done by capturing one's thought and deciding to work on it later, by analyzing the thought and seeing it as an unhealthy thought pattern, by interrogating the thought to see if it has any validity, and other techniques such as pinging oneself with a rubber wristband when unwanted thoughts occur. There is some controversy over whether attempting to suppress thoughts makes them even more intrusive (Smith, 2018). Nevertheless, thought stopping is a self-control procedure that is easily taught by paraprofessionals and is relatively easy for the secondarily traumatized person to enact.

*Progressive muscle relaxation* (PMR) (Jacobson, 1938) has a long history in the treatment of anxieties. It is a component of the SIT that is used in CISM, and it can be of value in managing the anxiety seen in secondary trauma. PMR is a self-control approach that rests upon the notion that an anxious mind seems unable to exist in a relaxed body. Relaxation approaches are so central in managing anxiety that they are found in CBT treatments of trauma, in yoga, and in meditation. PMR involves the tensing and relaxing of muscles in a fashion such that a muscle group is tensed for 5 s. It is then relaxed, and another muscle group is tensed and relaxed. A typical sequence might involve making fists with the hands, holding that for 5 s, and then letting go. The hands are then opened wide, splaying the fingers. This is held for 5 s and then released. Then the biceps are tensed without making fists and relaxed. One then moves to the triceps by attempting to bend the arms in the "wrong" direction. Facial muscles are then tensed followed by loosening of the muscles of the neck by turning one's head in one direction five times and then five times in the other direction. Shoulders are pulled inward and then pulled backward. Deep inhalation and exhalation expand and contract the muscles of the chest. The stomach is then distended followed by pulling it inward as if to touch the backbone. The heels are held a few inches off the floor, and the muscles of the calf and thigh muscles are tensed while curling the toes. With practice one develops the ability to relax more quickly and to also target those muscle groups that are most affected by anxiety. Relaxing imagery can also be paired with PMR to enhance its effectiveness. PMR is a skill that can be easily taught by those lacking professional mental health credentials.

## 13.3 Immersion in Nature

Immersion in nature is another highly effective approach to reducing the stresses associated with secondary traumatization. The heavy emotional burdens of caring for a family member, or the distress endured by first responders who continually deal with a variety of crises, or the "compassion fatigue" experienced by health-care providers can often be relieved by resorting to natural environments. The seemingly innate desire to commune with nature, natural environments, and lifelike processes has been labeled as "biophilia," and the term has been attributed to the naturalist and entomologist Edward O. Wilson (1984). There is a growing body of empirical research on the role that the natural environment plays in improving both physical and mental health (e.g., Van den Berg, 2017; van den Bosch & Depledge, 2015; White et al., 2017). Unfortunately, there is no precise methodological process to investigate how natural environments alleviate emotional distress of the type seen in secondary traumatization. Despite the lack of prescribed methodology, the health benefits of nature have been widely reported. In Japan, immersion in nature is a common practice that is used to alleviate life stressors whether due to job demands or family obligations. These excursions into nature are conducted by nonprofessionally trained guides. The term *shirin yoku* is translated as "forest bathing" and is a commonly employed stress reliever in Japan (Williams, 2017). In fact, nature immersion is widely used as a form of therapy and is defined as "an intervention with the aim to treat, hasten recovery, and/or rehabilitate … ill health … with the fundamental principle that the therapy involves plants, natural materials, and/or outdoor environments…" (Annerstedt & Wahrborg, 2011, p. 372).

It is difficult to design controlled studies that would effectively assess the degree to which nature positively impacts emotional well-being. Such studies entail random assignment, double-blind procedures, control groups, objective methodologies, and the use of psychometrically sound measures. One can imagine how difficult it would be to design such a study that would assess the impact of natural environments on health. Further, the more control one imposes on a study, the more likely it is that the study won't be relevant or generalizable to the "real world."

Waddell and Godderis (2005), for example, state that "What works in research settings may not be the same as what works in practice" (p. 60). Rather than pursue the experimentally controlled approach, what is done is that numerous studies, some well-controlled and some less so, are statistically combined in a meta-analysis, and one then examines "effect sizes." In a study of the impact of nature on health or in other such studies, an effect size would indicate the degree of change or the magnitude of impact that nature has upon health. In experimental research studies, effect sizes of .3 are small, .5 are medium, and .8 and higher are large. As will be described below, the effect size for the impact of natural environments on emotional adjustment is approximately .5, a medium effect size, and this degree of impact is considered both statistically significant and clinically meaningful.

Robbins (2020) reports on research findings based on 20,000 participants showing that immersion in nature has several positive impacts including reductions in anxiety and depression, reduced stress, enhanced mental clarity and focus, and enhanced creativity. These benefits also extend to the physical realm where reductions in blood pressure and reductions in stress hormones are shown, along with improved immune system response. These health benefits were associated with spending 2 h per week in local parks and natural environments. Two hours per week, whether condensed to one day or spread out over the week, was found to be the needed dosage or criterion. The health benefits did not accrue to spending less time in nature. Studies such as this are correlational and/or epidemiological in nature as it is exceedingly difficult to design controlled studies on the impact of natural environments.

The abundance of findings on the impact of the immersion in natural environments show there are clear potential benefits for those depleted by secondary traumatization and the accompanying exhaustion, depression, anxiety, and cynicism that is frequently associated with this disorder. The increase in urbanization of society unfortunately reduces the availability of abundant green spaces (Cox et al., 2017) and their health-promoting benefits. The increased time spent on screens and sedentary activities has only added to a reduction in exposure to natural environments (Hofferth, 2009).

Bowen and Neill (2013) conducted a meta-analysis of 197 studies of immersion in nature and in the process examined 2900 effect sizes among various measures. Recall that an effect size of .5 is medium and considered to be statistically and clinically meaningful. Across studies, individual psychotherapy shows an effect size of .68. The overall impact of nature program involvements found within this meta-analysis was approximately .5, a medium effect size. These authors also examined the effect size of there being no intervention, and it was found to be .08, and for alternative programs not involving nature, the effect size was .16. The authors found that age is an important factor in that older participants benefited more than children and adolescents from nature immersion. From this we might conclude that those adults typically engaged in first responder, family care, or health-care provider roles would benefit more than younger people.

Another large-scale meta-analysis was conducted by Neill (2003) in which participants were engaged in a variety of outdoor activities in natural environments.

Their responses on a variety of measures were systematically evaluated. Effect sizes on these measures varied from 1.04, a large effect size, to a small effect size of .24. Neill reports that larger effect sizes were from older participants engaged in longer programs run by organizations with established reputations. Neill's findings suggest that caution needs to be exercised when evaluating the impact of nature activities. There are several variables to be considered such as the activities in which one engages while in nature, the lengths of the programs, the ages of the participants, the initial levels of specific emotions such as anxiety and depression, levels of self-esteem, gender, and other factors. All these variables impact reported effect sizes.

In evaluating interventions such as the impact of immersion in nature on emotional and behavioral responses, such as those representing secondary trauma, it is often necessary to take a wide view and not limit oneself to only examining empirical studies involving random assignment and blinded methodologies. When these approaches are available, they should certainly be given priority as done by many professional organizations such as the American Psychological Association. However, in many instances such a level of control of independent variables is extremely difficult to achieve. Starting with observations such as those of Wilson (1984) who remarked on the attraction of humans to natural environments, to studies involving rural versus urban environments, to controlled studies and meta-analyses, and to examining combined findings over a period of decades, one is led inexorably to the conclusion that natural environments are health-producing and facilitate overall well-being. They alleviate psychological distress, promote mental clarity and focus, and result in physical health benefits. It is for these reasons that immersion in nature is recommended as a way of alleviating the emotional burdens of those silently suffering secondarily traumatized individuals whose commitment to others puts their own health and well-being at risk.

## 13.4 The Case of Sara

Sara is a 36-year-old caseworker for the Department of Social Services (DSS). While not formally trained in the law, she assists lawyers in preparation of cases involving the removal of children from homes in which they experienced various forms of physical, sexual, or emotional abuse and neglect. While she finds this work rewarding, she also remarked that it was "triggering" in that it reawakened memories of her own childhood difficulties.

Sara recognizes that her drive to help children may be fueled by her own abuse and the resulting desire to help children avoid what she endured. Sara is one of eight children, and she reports that in her childhood home there "simply wasn't enough attention to go around." Her mother reportedly worked as an elementary school teacher, and her father worked in construction. She recalls that during the period when she was 5–8 years of age, her father would "check" her underwear before she went to bed. He also did this to two of her other sisters. This behavior unnerved her especially when his checking also included genital touching, which was not an uncommon occurrence. She reports that even as a child she knew something was wrong with her father's behavior but was confused and saddened by it and did not mention it to her mother.

What added to Sara's distress was that in his mid-50 s her father began to develop a form of dementia, the specific nature of which was unknown to her at the time. Sara was subsequently thrust into becoming his ambivalent and dutiful caretaker. The most common form of dementia for people under 60 is frontotemporal lobar degeneration (Gupta, 2020), and it is likely that this is what afflicted Sara's father. This disorder involves a progressive loss of neurons in the frontal and/or temporal lobes and an impairment of memory, behavior, language, and movement. Sara states that the first symptoms that she saw her father display were forgetfulness, lack of coordination, and disorientation. Prior to his death, her father did not recognize Sara or other family members. "Although he was there physically, he was gone. He was a person I didn't know," claimed Sara. Working with her father was emotionally exhausting as he became increasingly unable to care for himself. Hand feeding and dealing with incontinence were chores that Sara grudgingly assumed. She felt compelled to be her father's caretaker even though other family members lent occasional assistance. It did not help matters that although she wanted to care for him and did so with characteristic diligence and commitment, she could not put out of her mind her father's inappropriate touching of her before bedtime. Sara loved her father despite her conflict over his bedtime rituals. All in all, he was a responsible father who took pride in his daughter's involvement in school and her commitment to bringing home excellent grades.

During the period of Sara's caretaking of her father, she found herself becoming so emotionally drained that when not caring for him or spending time at work, she would fall into an exhausted and non-rejuvenating sleep. This sequence became her life for 12 years. Care for her father, go to work and deal with troubling cases, come home, care for her father, and then exhaustedly lapse into sleep. What broke this cycle was that a colleague at work suggested that Sara adopt a puppy. At first the thought of having to care for another being caused Sara to reject this idea. Her friend persisted and brought Sara to a pet store in a nearby shopping mall. Sara saw several cute and affectionate puppies, but none grabbed her attention until she came upon a mini-Yorkie that was so small that she could hold it in one hand. This little dog immediately connected with Sara with its raw enthusiasm and excited barking. The little puppy tugged at Sara's heart. She felt an immediate connection that she described as "reciprocal love."

As things turned out, this little dog, whom she named Luka, grew to be all of three pounds as an adult. The need to care for Luka and to provide him with exercise required that Sara take a break from her preoccupations with her troubling work experiences and her commitments to her father. Luka needed Sara's attention and she began taking the little dog for walks at a local arboretum. She found that her time spent with this little, unconditionally loving dog, and their walks among the trees were rejuvenating. Her time in nature with Luka began to brighten her otherwise dreary and burdensome days. Realizing that she could enjoy herself, Sara began exploring other self-help options and initiated a self-directed program of progressive muscle relaxation and diaphragmatic breathing that she found on YouTube. Progressive muscle relaxation led to explorations of yoga and meditation practice, which she also found to be helpful in managing her abundant stress. Sara briefly began a period of counseling to further help her move away from her oppressive burdens but found that the need to make weekly appointments, as well as the time spent driving to these sessions, simply consumed too much of what little time she had for herself and her little Luka. As a result, Sara discontinued counseling but continued with her self-help activities.

Sara's case highlights how the serendipitous event of a friend's suggestion that she adopt a puppy snowballed into a series of healthy activities, all of which have been empirically shown to be health-promoting. The shared love between Sara and Luka was the bright spark that began moving Sara in a healthy direction. Realizing that relief from stress was within her reach, she pursued the self-help avenues of relaxation, yoga, and meditation. Her immersion in nature was profoundly rejuvenating for Sara and the exercise that Luka needed also provided Sara with the stress-relieving benefits of physical activity.

Sara hated to admit it to herself, but the eventual death of her father, sad though it was, was a relief for her. She no longer was required to care for a man who no longer recognized her and whose presence sparked uncomfortable feelings related to his inappropriate touching of her. Sara's multiple and empirically grounded self-help activities also helped her deal with the distressing cases she had to deal with at work. She found the child sexual abuse cases particularly distressing but also took comfort in the fact that removing these children from abusive homes provided them with an avenue of escape, one that she did not have for herself as a child. In all, Sara was able to make important changes in her life with no real involvement with professional health-care providers other than her brief stint with counseling. Sara's was a classic case of secondary traumatization brought on by the dual demands of caring for an increasingly disabled father and the stresses of the DSS cases that required her commitment to rescuing abused children. Involvement with her loving little Luka, her arboretum immersion, exercise, relaxation, yoga, and meditation all combined to lift Sara's spirits and to give her hope for a brighter day ahead. Sara has continued her health-promoting self-help activities, and although her work with DSS has become no less stressful, she is far better able to deal with her secondary traumatic stressors. When these stressors begin to build, Sara makes sure to plan additional trips to the green, nourishing environment of the local arboretum with her little companion.

## 13.5 Summary

The stressors and emotionally draining experiences of those who must care for an ailing family member, or the demands placed on health-care professionals and first responders, often precipitate a condition of emotional exhaustion identified as secondary or vicarious traumatization. This condition can often be ameliorated with nonprofessional or self-care interventions. Although there are specific exceptions, secondary trauma is not equivalent to what is seen in PTSD where one is directly accosted by terribly frightening events that are beyond one's control. In fact, all things considered, secondary trauma eventuates from experiences that are within one's control. Secondarily traumatized people have often chosen a profession or activity that demands so much of them that they are depleted and emotionally exhausted by the strains they encounter. PTSD is, in the main, a different diagnostic entity than secondary trauma. The PTSD sufferer has encountered an event or events that are so overwhelmingly disturbing and/or threatening that they are deeply and negatively altered. The PTSD sufferer no longer sees themselves in the same way as they used to. They have taken on many of the characteristics of a frightened animal, and they see their environment as potentially threatening. They have a profound sense of dread and wariness of others. These characteristics make treatment of them particularly difficult as therapists often unwittingly activate the PTSD sufferer's ever-present anxieties, and this commonly leads to leaving therapy or avoiding the process altogether. Secondary trauma, in most cases, does not require formal therapy but can benefit from paraprofessional interventions or self-initiated interventions.

Among these nonprofessional interventions are stress-debriefing activities. Stress debriefing, often referred to as critical incident stress debriefing (CISD), has a checkered history. There have been reports of secondarily and primarily traumatized individuals being made worse by interventions such as stress debriefing. It has been suggested that re-exposing people to traumatic experiences can exacerbate the negative impact of those experiences. A modification of CISD called critical incident stress management (CISM) has been reported to be more effective in reducing trauma experiences. The primary difference between these procedures is said to be that CISM incorporates a series of self-management procedures that are included within the rubric of stress inoculation training (SIT). SIT incorporates processes such as progressive muscle relaxation training, learning to activate this muscle relaxation in the face of stressors, diaphragmatic breathing, and learning to control one's negative thoughts and ruminations. The self-directed alteration of one's troubling thoughts is generically referred to as cognitive restructuring.

Another important nonprofessionally guided or self-guided activity that can help in reducing the negative impact of secondary trauma is immersion in nature. This chapter presents several empirical studies and meta-analyses that reveal compelling evidence for the beneficial effects of immersion in nature. In fact, "forest bathing" is a common approach to dealing with stressors like those seen in secondary trauma. It is an accepted practice in Japan that is either paraprofessionally guided or self-guided. Work stress, particularly the kind of stress that arises from giving of oneself emotionally is managed with weekend excursions into nature. Nature immersion such as walks through parks, wooded areas, and arboretums results in statistically and clinically meaningful reductions in stress and a sense of rejuvenation.

Finally, the case of Sara is presented, which highlights a common situation in which a family member must deal with another who is ailing. In this case dementia was the specific ailment. The case was complicated by the father's sexually inappropriate behaviors when Sara was a child and by the emotionally draining nature of her work. Nevertheless, Sara was immensely helped by her acquisition of a loving puppy and by a series of other activities including nature immersion, exercise, relaxation, yoga, and meditation. What this case highlights is that nonprofessional, self-directed care can be immensely uplifting and be of significant value in altering the emotionally draining and deadening impact of secondary traumatization.

# Chapter 14
# Key Takeaways

It has been the position of this book that while secondary trauma and PTSD may have some overlap, they are essentially different conditions that call for different forms of intervention. This view is contrary to that taken by some investigators in the secondary trauma field who assert that the two conditions are "nearly identical." Several of these investigators describe secondary trauma as involving "compassion fatigue" and emotional exhaustion arising from the giving of oneself in the service of others. While this giving of oneself may be the cornerstone of secondary trauma, it is not a causal factor in the development of PTSD. Instead, PTSD is a reaction to extremely threatening situations, and the consequences of these threats can alter a person, sometimes for their entire lives. Rather than exhibiting the symptoms of being exhausted or drained as in secondary traumatization, the PTSD sufferer evidences a profoundly altered view of their environment and of themselves. They often view their environment with suspicion, fear, and distrust. Similarly, their view of themselves has also changed. They frequently report being dehumanized by their traumatic experience, and some see themselves as acting as frightened animals. To claim that secondary trauma and PTSD are nearly alike or identical is simply unwarranted.

Terms such as vicarious trauma, secondary trauma, empathic strain, compassion fatigue, shared trauma, and the like may have some nuanced differences; however, several authors (e.g., Phipps & Byrne, 2003; Sexton, 1999) see these terms as essentially interchangeable. It is for this reason that the general terms *secondary trauma* or *secondary traumatic stress disorder* have been used to encompass all of them in this book. Secondarily traumatized people may feel "burnt out," but burnout can also apply to situations not involving dealing with others who are distressed. It can be used to describe a reaction to employment situations that are so physically and emotionally demanding that one is simply drained and exhausted. As a result, burnout, although used in the secondary trauma literature, can be the outcome of situations that do not involve dealing with distressed or traumatized individuals.

© The Author(s), under exclusive license to Springer Nature Switzerland AG 2023

R. W. Motta, *Secondary Trauma*, https://doi.org/10.1007/978-3-031-44308-4_14

The primary sources of secondary trauma that have been addressed in this book are those arising in *the family* where a caretaker becomes emotionally drained by aiding a member who is either traumatized or severely ailing in some way. Another group that has been focused on is *first responders* such as firefighters, police officers, EMTs, paramedics, disaster response workers, and other community helpers whose jobs involve the assurance of public safety. First responders often find themselves secondarily traumatized and exhausted in the efforts to help others in distress. *Professional caregivers* are another group who are regularly secondarily traumatized. Mental health therapists, medical doctors, nurses, and other health-care providers who give of themselves in treating those who are emotionally and/or physically distressed or incapacitated are frequently overwhelmed by the demands of the care they provide. The constant giving of help to those in physical or emotional distress can result in becoming emotionally depleted and debilitated and in some cases acquiring the same fears and concerns of those they treat. There are many other groups who experience secondary trauma, including children and adolescents, and while their concerns are addressed in this book, the primary focus is on family members, first responders, and professional caregivers.

## 14.1 Perspectives on Interventions for Secondary Trauma

Another position that is taken in this book that may be at odds with the views of some writers involves interventions for secondary trauma. If one views secondary trauma and PTSD as being nearly identical, it follows, according to some writers, that the treatment of these two disorders should also be highly similar. This position appears at odds with the nature of the two diagnostic groups. They are hardly identical. In fact, Bercier and Maynard (2015), following a review of four thousand studies found no compelling evidence that secondary trauma should be treated in the same manner as PTSD. They also found no evidence, given the low quality of existing studies, that would strongly point to the value of any specific intervention being more effective than others. The "gold standard" for treating PTSD is said to be cognitive-behavioral psychotherapy (CBT), which often includes prolonged exposure (PE) whereby PTSD sufferers are repeatedly presented with the traumatic stimuli and with their recalled reactions to these stimuli until they become inured to trauma stimuli. The primary focus of CBT is the replacement of dysfunctional and maladaptive cognitions with more reasonable and objective views. CBT and PE interventions aim to right thoughts and behaviors that are dysfunctional and that impair overall well-being. While there may be many other methods of treating PTSD that can be found in the literature, CBT interventions for trauma disorders are reflective of the zeitgeist in the USA and much of the world.

The question that needs to be asked is do those who experience secondary trauma have similar disturbances of thought, emotion, and behavior as those with PTSD? When one examines those suffering from secondary trauma, one finds that there is little that is illogical in the thinking processes of these individuals. They are often emotionally burnt out and drained from what they do and may experience accompanying anxiety and depression over the stressors they endure, but their thinking is not illogical or maladaptive like that seen in PTSD. Secondarily traumatized people may be depressed over the nature of their work and have anxiety over the thought of having to confront their next demanding case or situation, but this is not illogical or maladaptive thinking. In fact, it is reasonable. Those experiencing secondary trauma require avenues of relief from their stress. This relief can take the form of seeking out the company of colleagues, family, and friends, seeking out relaxing or distracting activities, and engaging in health practices like yoga, meditation, and the like. But these activities are not formal types of "therapy" as is often required in the treatment of PTSD. It may be true that in certain extremely distressing situations, the family member, first responder, or health-care professional may require formal psychotherapy, but in general, secondary trauma does not call upon this type of intervention. Before delving into why specific interventions are of value, a more fundamental question should be addressed, as follows.

## 14.2 Why Do We Have Secondary Trauma Reactions in the First Place?

This is a reasonable question. Of what value is secondary trauma in terms of the evolution of humans (and, in fact, several other animals)? Consider what things would be like if we had no concern for others. We would not be secondarily traumatized because we would not be impacted by the distress of others. We would be able to watch others suffer without undue concern. Perhaps we would be sociopaths whose defining characteristic is a lack of conscience and a lack of caring for anyone other than ourselves (Stout, 2005). The stance of emotional coldness to the pain of others would probably impede species survival. Our concern for the welfare of others induces us to help, and this often means assisting others and thereby helping ourselves to survive. There is safety in numbers. It is likely that the ability to experience secondary trauma helps in supporting the survival of our own species. We need each other to assure our own viability as a species.

The inclination to be concerned with and impacted by the emotional state of others appears to develop at an early age. Children less than 1 year of age have been found to display an emotional reaction to the expressions of upset in adults. Even primate studies show that monkeys will go without food if doing so prevents another monkey from being shocked. Observations such as these have been replicated and suggest that we are "hardwired" to react to the distress of others and this wiring works to ensure species survival. Research on "mirror neurons" shows that primates and humans often respond not only to the actions of others but to their intentions to act. In addition to being hardwired, there is little doubt that there is a socialization component to the potential development of secondary trauma responses. We are socialized to be concerned with the welfare of others. But the mirror neuron studies and the primate studies suggest that more than social learning is involved. The capacity to be concerned with the welfare of others appears to be part of our biological-genetic and social heritage.

## 14.3 Secondary Trauma and Treatment in Children

Secondary trauma reactions are seen in children just as they are in adults. When a child sees that their parents are in distress, they too react with distress. A perspective that has been presented in this book is that children may be reacting to a sense of loss. This loss is of the parent or caretaker that they once knew. The caretaker may have been previously supportive, comforting, and loving and now, because of some form of stress, appears remote, unavailable, or preoccupied with issues that the child is often unaware of. It was noted that in situations that are threatening to the family, the children will often react more to parental and caretaker reactions than to the actual family threat. When Hurricane or "super storm" Sandy hit the East Coast of the USA in 2012, children appeared to be less fearful of the rising tides and torrential rain than they were of seeing their parents being fearful and upset. The same phenomenon was reported in the bombing of London in World War II. The fear shown by parents had a greater negative impact on children than did the bombings themselves. Children were unnerved by the loss or change they saw in their parents and caretakers. The reassuring and comforting caretaker now appeared threatened and fearful, and as a result the children became fearful. A similar situation was seen in the kibbutzim in Israel where the reaction of parents had more of an impact on children than the surrounding battles.

So how are the secondary trauma reactions of these children addressed or treated? They are generally not treated with CBT or some other form of child therapy, but rather, children regain their sense of normalcy and balance when they are reassured and provided with information. When they see their caretakers resume their positions as protectors, providers of nurturance, and sources of reassurance, then the children experience a reduction in anxiety and dread. They feel that the world they knew and grown accustomed to has been restored. Their parents and caretakers have resumed the roles that the children are familiar with, and as a result their anxieties and sense of loss are quelled. Therapy in the traditional sense is not needed here because there are no cognitive, emotional, or behavioral dysfunctions that are out of sync with reality. When parents and caretakers become threatened, the security and safety of children are also threatened. These are normal responses, not responses requiring psychotherapy. What we see here is that secondary trauma reactions may require something other than formal psychotherapy. For secondarily traumatized children, a return to the familiar environment involving their parents and caretakers is what is called for.

## 14.4 Secondary Trauma and Treatment in Adults

Adults who experience secondary trauma reactions often find themselves in the roles of caretakers and protectors. The most frequently occurring source of secondary trauma in adults is being in the role of providing support to an ailing, impaired, or traumatized family member. The needy family member may have an impairing and painful physical ailment or may perhaps be suffering from an emotional disorder or a neurologically based ailment that alters their thinking and perception. Regardless of the nature of the family member's problem, the caretaker may become "infected" by that person's distress, and the distress therefore becomes a "shared trauma." As a result, the caretaker eventually may become emotionally drained and depleted in their efforts to provide care. This is a classic example of what has been referred to as compassion fatigue.

Police officers, firefighters, EMTs, paramedics, disaster relief workers, and many others whose jobs entail the provision of public safety may also become traumatized by witnessing the plight of those in distress. At times, the trauma of first responders can become intense enough to result in PTSD, but it is unclear whether they are more impaired by their trauma experiences than other care providers. "Although first responders are among the most trauma-exposed groups, a large gap remains between the evidence on the development and management of their mental health and what is known about other trauma-exposed populations" (Bryant, 2021, p. 198). Their efforts to provide care, safety, and support can be so emotionally depleting, as they go from one emergency to the next, that a probable diagnosis of secondary trauma is often warranted. These people need relief, and like the children noted above, relief comes less from "therapy" than from more common, everyday, stress-relieving interventions.

In addition to adult caregivers and first responders, professional care providers are also one of the populations vulnerable to the development of secondary trauma. This group includes, but is not necessarily limited to, mental health-care providers, and physical health-care personnel, such as medical doctors, nurses, physician assistants, and occupational and physical therapists. These individuals are often involved on a one-to-one basis with those who are suffering from a variety of mental, emotional, and physical ailments. Like the other groups, they are vicariously traumatized by their exposure to a series of suffering individuals. Therapists can sometimes acquire the fears and trauma responses of those they treat. At times their secondary traumatic stress becomes so draining and so burdensome that they find leaving their profession as the only way of alleviating their distress. Elevated suicide rates among health-care providers have been reported.

One of the many contributors that magnify their potential secondary traumatization is their self-imposed inability to escape. While the inability to escape may seem counterintuitive, as nothing prevents them from leaving their professions, it is their commitment, and identity that can serve as a roadblock to leaving. Health-care providers are professionals who often have a deeply ingrained identification with their profession. They are constrained from leaving their stressful work by an identity that mandates the alleviation of distress of others. It has been noted that trauma reactions are magnified by the inability to escape. When escape is possible, the probability of developing a trauma reaction is lessened. Health-care providers experience a self-imposed commitment and dedication to their work such that they will often place their own well-being in a position that is secondary to the well-being of those they treat. In fact, this is often seen as the mark of a "real" dedicated provider. It is in this way that their avenues of escape are blocked and their chances of being secondarily or vicariously traumatized (McCann & Pearlman, 1990) are enhanced. This group, like the others noted above, requires intervention and treatment, but in most instances this assistance does not entail formal psychotherapy as their problems have far less to do with psychopathology than emotional depletion, exhaustion, and absorption of emotional distress originating from the traumas they treat.

## 14.5 Treatment Specifics: Family Therapy, CISD, and CISM

There are perhaps innumerable ways of alleviating the distress of secondary trauma. Those that have been covered have received some level of empirical support, but there are doubtless others that are not covered, which are probably effective and which may or may not be supported by empirical studies. Those that have been addressed in this book have been grouped under the rubric of "structural interventions" to distinguish them from psychotherapeutic interventions such as various cognitive-behavioral therapies, psychoanalysis, behavior therapy, nondirective therapy, and the like.

Among these structural interventions is family therapy (e.g., Figley & Figley, 2009). Family therapy has been advocated by those who maintain that families can be both the source of secondary trauma and a resource for treating this disorder. Given the contagious nature of traumatic experiences, families of the secondarily traumatized individual are impacted, but they can also serve as a source of support in helping that individual manage their distress.

Self-care treatments for the secondarily traumatized have been advocated by several authors (e.g., Gilbert-Eliot, 2020; Molnar et al., 2017; Norcross, 2000; Phipps & Byrne, 2003). An amalgam of self-care strategies has been suggested by these authors including mindfulness-based stress reduction, self-awareness training, human contact, counseling, stimulus control, avoidance of self-blame and wishful thinking, diversification of activities, restructuring one's job responsibilities, scheduling time off, debriefing, psychoeducation, seeking training in additional job skills, stress management skills, and others.

Nonprofessional or paraprofessional interventions have also been proposed. Among these are critical incident stress debriefing (CISD) (Mitchell, 1983) and critical incident stress management (CISM) (Mitchell & Everly, 2000). CISD has something of a checkered past in that it has often been conducted as a one-shot intervention that takes place shortly after trauma exposure, although it may not have been initially intended as a one-shot procedure. The intention of implementing the intervention shortly after trauma exposure is that by doing so, the traumatic experiences do not have the opportunity to become consolidated as might occur with the passage of time. Unfortunately, what has been found in several studies is that instituting an intervention that entails a detailed recall of events and equally detailed descriptions of one's emotional reactions to those events heightens emotional arousal and, in that way, may make matters worse. Follow-up studies of CISD have, on several occasions, revealed a worsening of trauma symptoms. A variant of CISD, CISM has shown more promising effects. CISM is not a one-shot intervention but often involves a follow-up of those who are treated. The follow-up includes additional care if needed. Also included in CISM is the provision of self-control procedures. These self-control procedures are part of a package referred to as stress inoculation training (SIT) (Michenbaum, 1985) and include activities such as progressive muscle relaxation, diaphragmatic breathing, and cognitive restructuring, that is, the alteration of dysfunctional cognitions. While it may be unclear as to whether the benefits of CISM are due to follow-up or due to the use of SIT components, CISM has been empirically shown to be a potentially valuable intervention that can be used by first responder organizations and other groups designed to arm participants against the potential negative impacts of trauma exposure.

## 14.6 Social Support, Exercise, Mindfulness, and Yoga

There are a series of interventions for secondary trauma that can be either self-initiated or facilitated by paraprofessionals. Social support is one of these interventions. Social support can be a formally structured and scheduled activity that is initiated by professional organizations or a far more casual effort by those impacted by secondary trauma to seek solace in the company of others. Overall empirical findings show that social support has a beneficial impact on alleviating secondary trauma and the feelings of isolation that may be fostered by secondary trauma experiences. There are studies that show, however, that too much discussion of traumatic experiences or too much personal revealing can have detrimental effects. Nevertheless, human beings are social animals, and we benefit from the company of others who may or may not have had similar experiences.

Exercise has shown itself to be an empirically validated intervention for dealing with trauma reactions, anxiety, and depression. There is considerable debate as to why this might be the case, and several hypotheses have been advanced. Despite the existence of these hypotheses, there is no universally agreed-upon reason for the efficacy of exercise in alleviating dysphoric states, despite the clear evidence that it does. One provocative explanation for the effectiveness of exercise is the bodymind view of Pert (1999) in which body and mind states are not seen as separate but rather as an integrated entity. Exercise is then seen as beneficial because it enhances this hypothesized bodymind entity. Regardless of speculations as to why exercise is beneficial in dealing with secondary trauma, it is probably best to view it as a validated intervention for this disorder and its accompanying anxiety and depression. There are times when a particular treatment or intervention is shown to be effective, but the underlying reason for its effectiveness is unknown. It took decades between the discovery of the antibiotic properties of aspirin by Alexander Fleming in 1928 and the elucidation of its mechanisms in 1995 (van der Kolk, 2014). Similarly, we may not be entirely certain as to why exercise is beneficial for traumatized states, but abundant evidence shows that it is.

Mindfulness meditation is particularly beneficial for managing the mind wanderings seen in those who have experienced trauma. Those suffering from secondary trauma often find that their thoughts drift to disturbing events they have encountered. Meditation involves intentional focusing of attention, and as such it works as a counter to the default mode of mind wandering. In practicing meditation, one learns to gain control over unwanted, intrusive thoughts by intentionally attending to the present moment. Empirical studies and meta-analyses support the utility of mindfulness in offsetting the negative impact of various trauma encounters. Nevertheless, mindfulness meditation is not a panacea for two reasons. First, it requires a high level of discipline to practice it daily. In a sense, it is somewhat like exercise in that it must be an ongoing and continual practice for it to have value. The second caveat is that mindfulness meditation is not easy to do. Even the most experienced of meditators are engaged in a constant battle during the practice of meditating with wanderings of the mind and returning to the present moment. Despite these two cautions, overall findings show that mindfulness meditation can be of real value in dealing with and reducing the negative impact of secondary trauma by reducing the intrusion of disturbing and unwanted trauma-related thoughts and preoccupations.

Yoga, like mindfulness, can be conducted in organized groups or done on one's own through apps, YouTube, or other forms of video presentation. People who have experienced trauma of various kinds often deal with it by pushing away unwanted memories or separating themselves from these disturbing remembrances. Yoga, which has been in existence for approximately five thousand years and is practiced in numerous different forms today, is an activity that emphasizes integration. Whereas trauma often involves separation of thoughts and feelings, yoga counters this tendency with the practice of a focal integration of body and mind. Engaging in postures or asanas requires a mental focus on body positions and body sensations, so it induces the practitioner to engage in integration processes. One might critique yoga in that while engaging in the practice of asanas, the mind might wander to disturbing and unwanted memories. However, overall empirical findings from both individual studies and meta-analyses reveal acceptable effect sizes showing that yoga beneficially impacts various forms of trauma along with anxiety and depression. The sheer popularity and accessibility of yoga have made it a viable trauma intervention that is often used with uniformed service organizations and by secondarily traumatized individuals in general.

## 14.7 Animals and Natural Environments

The presence of animals can be effective in ameliorating the negative impact of secondary trauma. Some authors (e.g., Hajar, 2015) report that animals have a unique capability to reduce stress, reduce anxiety and depression, encourage exercise and playfulness, and serve as an excellent distractor, all the while providing unbounded and unconditional love and affection. The historic record shows that animals have had a beneficial relationship with humans that dates back thousands of years BCE. The unconditional love, support, and acceptance shown by animals, particularly dogs, can be a significant stress reliever to traumatized individuals.

Dogs have played two roles in regard to trauma-related stress. The first role is that of a loving, unconditionally accepting companion whose presence combats feelings of isolation and whose needs for exercise and feeding can draw the traumatized individual out of their reclusive and avoidant inclinations while distracting them from obsessive, trauma-related cognitions and preoccupations. The unconditional love dogs provide draws forth a similar response from their caretaker. It is difficult not to return the affection of an unconditionally accepting and loving dog. The second role is that of a service animal. Controlled studies show that dogs can engage in specific activities to help those who are traumatized, such as waking them when they are having nightmares, encouraging physical activities, alerting them to situations that the caretaker may see as threatening, reminding caretakers to take medication, and serving as a physical barrier to potentially anxiety-provoking encounters.

The beneficial impact of animals encompasses a whole array of animals including, but not limited to, cats, horses, pigs, hamsters, rabbits, and many other animals, some of which are not known to be particularly attached to humans, such as fish and reptiles. The care needs of fish and reptiles can elicit compassionate responses from humans. There have been a series of studies involving horses and their beneficial impact on both youngsters and adults who have experienced trauma and other disorders such as ADHD, Alzheimer's, depression, anxiety, autism, and personality problems. Programs of therapeutic horseback riding have been instituted to help military service members who are suffering from assorted traumas including PTSD (e.g., Lanning et al., 2018). It is unclear why therapeutic horseback riding would be effective in reducing PTSD, loneliness, and depression to a significant degree while enhancing perceptions of self-efficacy and self-worth, but these have been the findings from randomized, controlled studies even after a period of only 3 weeks. Even "plush" or stuffed animals have been found to have a positive impact on residents in eldercare facilities and hospitals.

Animals appear to bring out our compassion and inclination to provide care. It is unclear why this is the case. It is likely that their inability to plan and scheme allows us to see their innocence and to elicit our trust and care. A client of mine put it simply: "Animals humanize us." Those suffering from the negative sequelae of secondary traumatization will often find engagement with animals to be both distracting and providing the essential emotional sustenance that has been drained from them.

A final "intervention" that has been shown to alleviate both everyday stressors and those arising from various forms of traumatic encounters is immersion in natural environments. The term *biophilia*, or our attraction to nature, has been attributed to the renowned entomologist E.O. Wilson (1984). He noted that human beings feel at home in natural environments and that nature has health-producing effects. The Japanese regularly practice *shinrin-yoku* or forest bathing as a common stress reliever. This involves either organized or individually initiated immersions into forests, parks, arboretums, or other natural settings. Both empirical and anecdotal evidence attests to the stress relief found in nature.

Meta-analytic studies involving tens of thousands of participants have shown that immersion in nature yields effect sizes of about .5, a medium effect size, in reducing negative affective states and enhancing perceptions of efficacy and self-worth. Medium effect sizes are both clinically and statistically meaningful. Other studies show that well-organized nature immersion programs with older participants show even larger effect sizes. One author (Robbins, 2020) contended that there is empirical support for the requirement of 2 hours per week in nature being the minimum needed to have significant reductions in anxiety, depression, and of course the exhaustion that characterizes secondary trauma reactions.

It is in some ways unfortunate that as a society we seem to be moving away from nature. We are increasingly drawn to cities and away from rural settings and to screens and virtual realities in the place of real-life encounters. In doing so we are increasingly separating ourselves from the health-producing benefits of exposure to nature. The toxins that are unwittingly pumped into our natural environment and the increasing destruction of these environments in the name of "development" have only served to further diminish this natural and valuable stress reliever. While it may be difficult to design studies that are held to the highest standards, that is, double-blind, placebo-controlled studies and randomized controlled trials (RCTs) when attempting to evaluate the impact of nature on psychological and physical health, the studies and meta-analyses that have been conducted show that it is important that we not overlook immersion in nature as a resource for managing secondary trauma.

## 14.8 Future Directions

A good deal of further research is needed so that we are better able to understand the complex processes that bring about secondary trauma. This requires a careful study of not only individual client characteristics and their histories, but also a careful evaluation of what specific factors within secondarily traumatizing environments may be more impairing than others. Further research into interventions is also needed. This area of study is particularly important as there is a virtual absence of investigations that compare one intervention to others as a way of finding what the most effective means of treating secondary traumatization is. There has been a good deal of high-quality research in primary trauma and PTSD, and yet even here additional studies are needed particularly in better understanding of comparative treatment effectiveness. The area of secondary trauma is in its infancy, and yet when one considers the "contagious" nature of trauma, it is highly likely that there are many more individuals suffering from the impact of secondary than primary trauma. Humans are certainly social animals, and it is this characteristic that creates a fertile environment for the development of secondary traumatization. It is hoped that additional studies will help us to both identify and effectively treat those secondarily traumatized individuals who are most in need.

# References


Abdill, M. N., & Juppe, D. (2005). *Pets in therapy: Animal assisted activities in health care facilities*. Idyll Arbor.

Adams, K. B., Matto, H. C., & Harrington, D. (2001). The traumatic stress institute belief scale as a measure of vicarious trauma in a national sample of clinical social workers. *Families in Society: The Journal of Contemporary Human Services, 82*(4), 363–371.

Adams, R. E., Figley, C. R., & Boscarino, J. A. (2008). The compassion fatigue scale: Its use with social workers following urban disaster. *Research in Social Work Practice, 18*(3), 238–250.

Alfermann, D., & Stoll, O. (Eds.). (2005). *Sportpsychologie: EinLehrbuch in 12 Lekionen* [Sports psychology: A textbook in 12 lessons]. Meyer & Meyer Verlag.

Altchiler, L., & Motta, R. W. (1997). Effects of aerobic and non-aerobic exercise on anxiety, depression, and job satisfaction. *Journal of Clinical Psychology, 50*, 829–840.

American Association of Retired Persons (AARP) and National Alliance for Caregiving. (2020). https://doi.org/10.26419/ppi.00103.003.

American Psychiatric Association (1980). *Diagnostic and statistical manual of mental Disorders* (3rd ed.). Washington DC: Author.

American Psychiatric Association. (2013). *Diagnostic and statistical manual of mental Disorders* (5th ed.). Author.

Anderson, A. R., Keyes, G. M., & Jobes, D. A. (2016). Understanding and treating suicidal Riskin young children. *Practice Innovations, 1*, 3–19.

Annerstedt, M., & Wahrborg, P. (2011). Nature-assisted therapy: Systematic review of controlled and observational studies. *Scandinavian Journal of Public Health, 39*, 371–388.

Ash, M. J., Walker, E. R., DiClemente, R. J., Florian, M. P., Palmer, P. K., Wehrmeyer, K., Negi, L. T., Grant, G. H., Raison, C. L., & Mascaro, J. S. (2021, October–December). Compassion meditation training for hospital chaplain residents: A pilot study. *Journal of Health Care Chaplaincy, 27*(4), 191–206.

Baird, K., & Kracen, A. C. (2006). Vicarious traumatization and secondary traumatic stress: A research synthesis. *Counseling Psychology Quarterly, 19*, 181–188.

Bandura, A. (1997). *Self-efficacy: The exercise of control*. Freeman.

Banks, K., Newman, E., & Saleem, J. (2015). An overview of the research on mindfulness-based interventions for treating symptoms of posttraumatic stress disorder: A systematic review. *Journal of Clinical Psychology, 71*, 935–963.

Bauhoff, S. (2011). Systematic self-report bias in health data: Impact on estimatingcross-sectional and treatment effects. *Health Services and Outcomes Research Methodology, 11*(1), 44–53.

Beach, S. R., Schulz, R., Donovan, H., & Rosland, A.-M. (2021). Family caregiving during the COVID-19 pandemic. *The Gerontologist*. https://doi.org/10.1093/geront/gnab049


© The Editor(s) (if applicable) and The Author(s), under exclusive license to Springer Nature Switzerland AG 2023

R. W. Motta, *Secondary Trauma*, https://doi.org/10.1007/978-3-031-44308-4

Beaton, R., & Murphy, S. (1993). Sources of occupational stress among firefighters/EMTs and firefighter/paramedics and correlations with job-related outcomes. *Prehospital and Disaster Medicine, 8*, 140–150.

Beaton, R., & Murphy, S. (1995). Working with people in crisis: Research implications. In C. R. Figley (Ed.), *Compassion fatigue: Coping with secondary traumatic stress disorder in those who treat the traumatized* (pp. 51–81). Routledge.

Beck, M. (2010, December 21). Beside Freud's couch, a chow named Jofi. *The Wall Street Journal.* Retrieved from https://www.wsj.com/articles/SB10001424052748703886904576031630124087362.

Beckman, S. (2015). *Secondary traumatic stress and posttraumatic growth: Risk and protective factors among American Red Cross disaster responder and disaster mental health workers* (Unpublished doctoral dissertation). University of Minnesota.

Beetz, A., Schoffman, I., Girgensohn, R., Brass, R., & Ernst, C. (2019). Positive effects of a short-term dog-assisted intervention with soldiers with post-traumatic stress disorder-A pilot study. *Frontiers of Veteran Science, 6*, 170. *eCollection* 2019. https://doi.org/10.3389/fvets.2019.00170

Benedek, D. M., & Wynn, G. H. (2016). *Complementary and alternative medicine for PTSD.* Oxford University Press.

Benedek, D. M., Fulleron, C., & Ursano, R. J. (2007). First responders: Mental health consequences of natural and human made disasters for public health and public safety workers. *Annual Review of Public Health, 28*, 55–68.

Benson, H. (1975). *The relaxation response*. Morrow.

Bentley, M. A., Crawford, J. M., Wilkins, J. R., Fernandez, A. R., & Studnek, J. R. (2013). An assessment of depression, anxiety, and stress among nationally certified EMS professionals. *Prehospital Emergency Care, 17*(3), 330–338. https://doi.org/10.3109/10903127.2012.761307

Bercier, M. L., & Maynard, B. R. (2015). Interventions for secondary traumatic stress with mental health workers: A systematic review. *Research in Social Work, 25*(1), 81–89.

Berger, R., & Gelkkopf, M. (2011). An intervention for reducing secondary traumatization and improving professional self-efficacy in well baby clinic nurses following war and terror: A random control group trial. *International Journal of Nursing Studies, 48*, 601–610.

Bernstein, E. E., & McNally, R. J. (2017). Acute aerobic exercise hastens emotional recovery from a subsequent stressor. *Health Psychology, 36*(6), 560–567.

Bober, T., & Regehr. (2006). Strategies for reducing secondary or vicarious trauma: Do they work. *Brief Treatment and Crisis Intervention, 6*(1), 1–9.

Bos, M. G., Schuijer, J., Lodestijn, F., Beckers, T., & Kindt, M. (2014). Stress enhances reconsolidation of declarative memory. *Psychoneuro, 46*, 102–113.

Boscarino, J. A., Adams, R. E., Figley, C. R., Galea, S., & Foa, E. B. (2006). Fear of terrorism and preparedness in New York City 2 years after the attacks: Implications for disaster planning and research. *Journal of Public Health Management and Practice, 12*, 505–513.

Bosoglu, M., Livanou, M., & Crnobaric, C. (2007). Torture vs. other cruel, inhuman anddegrading treatment: Is the distinction real or apparent? *Achieves of General Psychiatry, 64*, 277–285.

Bowen, D. J., & Neill, J. T. (2013). A meta-analysis of adventure therapy outcomes and moderators. *Open Psychology Journal, 6*, 28–53.

Bowlby, J. (1982). *Attachment and loss, Vol. 1: Attachment.* Basic Books (Original work published 1968).

Boyer, B., Bubel, D., Jacobs, S. R., Knolls, M., Harwell, V. D., Goscicka, M., et al. (2002). Posttraumatic stress in women with breast cancer and their daughters. *The American Journal of Family Therapy, 30*, 328–338.

Brooks, S. K., Dunn, R., Sage, C. A., Amlot, R., Greenberg, N., & Rubin, G. J. (2015). Risk and resilience factors affecting the psychological wellbeing of individuals deployed in humanitarian relief roles after a disaster. *Journal of Mental Health, 24*(6), 385–413.

Brooks, S. K., Dunn, R., Amlot, R., Greenberg, N., & Rubin, G. J. (2016). Social and occupational factors associated with psychological stress and disorder among disaster responders: A systematic review. *BMC Psychology, 4*(18), 1–13.

Brough, P. (2005). A comparative investigation of the predictors of work-related psychological well-being within police, fire and ambulance workers. *New Zealand Journal of Psychology, 34*(2), 127–134.
Bryant, R. A. (2021). *Treating PTSD in first responders: A guide to serving those who serve.* American Psychological Association.
Bryant, R. A., Moulds, M. L., Mastrodomenico, J., Hopwood, S., Felmingham, K., & Nixon, R. D. V. (2007). Who drops out of treatment for posttraumatic stress disorder? *Clinical Psychologist, 11*, 13–15.
Bushman, B. (Ed.). (2017). *ACSM's completed guide to fitness & health* (2nd ed.). Human Kinetics.
Büssing, A., Michalsen, A., Khalsa, S. B., Telles, S., & Sherman, K. J. (2012). Effects of yoga on mental and physical health: A short summary of reviews. *Evidence-Based Complementary and Alternative Medicine: eCAM, 2012*, 165410. https://doi.org/10.1155/2012/165410
Butler, D., & Moseley, G. L. (2015). *The explain pain protectometer handbook (8315).* NOI Group.
Calhoun, L. G., & Tedeschi, R. G. (2013). *Posttraumatic growth in clinical practice.* Routledge.
Campbell, S. (2021). *The effects of secondary trauma on executive functioning in law enforcement officers* (Unpublished doctoral dissertation). The Chicago School of Professional Psychology.
Catherall, D. R. (1992). *Back from the brink: A family guide to overcoming traumatic stress.* Bantam Books.
Caringella, S. (2009). *Addressing rape reform in law and practice.* Columbia University Press: New York.
Center for Mindfulness in Medicine, Health Care, and Society. (n.d.). *History of MBSR.* Retrieved from https://www.umassmed.edu/cfm/mindfulness-based-programs/mbsr-courses/about-mbsr/history-of-mbsr/
Centers for Disease Control and Prevention, National Center for Injury Prevention and Control. Web-based Injury Statistics Query and Reporting System (WISQARS), fatal injury reports, 2014, for national, regional, and states (restricted). Available at www.cdc.gov/ncipc/wisqars
Cohen, S., & Wills, T. A. (1985). Stress, social support, and the buffering hypothesis. *Psychological Bulletin, 98*(2), 310–357.
Collins, R. (2008). *Violence: A micro-sociological theory.* Princeton University Press.
Cox, D. T. C., Hudson, H. L., Shanahan, D. F., Fuller, R. A., & Gaston, K. J. (2017). The rarity of direct experiences of nature in an urban population. *Landscape and Urban Planning, 160*, 79–84.
Craft, L. L. (2005). Exercise and clinical depression: Examining two psychological mechanisms. *Psychology of Sport and Exercise, 6*(2), 151–171.
Craft, L. L., & Perna, F. M. (2004). The benefits of exercise for the clinically depressed. *The Primary Care Companion to the Journal of Clinical Psychiatry, 6*(3), 104–111.
Cramer, H., Lauche, R., Langhorst, J., & Dobos, G. (2013). Yoga for depression: A systematic review and meta-analysis. *Depression and Anxiety, 30*, 1068–1083.
Cummings, E. M., Zahn-Waxler, C., & Radke-Yarrow, M. (1981). Young children's responses to expressions of anger and affections by others in the family. *Child Development, 52*(4), 1274–1282.
Curley, T., Campbell, A. A., Doyle, J. N., & Freeze, S. M. (2021). First responders' perceptions of the presence of support canines in the workplace. *Journal of Police and Criminal Psychology.* https://doi.org/10.1007/s/11896-021-09477-4
da Silva, T. L., Ravindran, L. N., & Ravindran, A. V. (2009). Yoga in the treatment of moodand anxiety disorders: A review. *Asian Journal of Psychiatry, 2*, 6–16.
Damasio, A. (2010). *Self comes to mind: Constructing the conscious brain.* Vintage Books.
Danieli, Y. E. (1998). *International handbook of multigenerational legacies of trauma.* Plenum.
Daniels, R. (2002). *Coming to America: A history of immigration and ethnicity in American life* (2nd ed.). Harper Collins.
Dass, R. (1978). *Be here now.* Harmony.
Deahl, M. (2000). Psychological debriefing: Controversy and challenge. *New Zealand Journal of Psychiatry, 34*, 929–939.

DeBoer, L. B., Powers, M. B., Utschig, A. C., Otto, M. W., & Smits, J. A. (2012). Exploring exercise as an avenue for the treatment of anxiety disorders. *Expert Review of Neurotherapeutics, 12*, 1011–1022.

Diaz, A. B., & Motta, R. W. (2008). The effects of an aerobic exercise program on posttraumatic stress disorder symptom severity in adolescents. *International Journal of Emergency Mental Health, 10*, 49–59.

Dick, A. M., Niles, B. L., Street, A. E., DiMartino, D. M., & Mitchell, K. S. (2014). Examining mechanisms of change in a yoga intervention for women: The influence of mindfulness, psychological flexibility, and emotional regulation on PTSD symptoms. *Journal of Clinical Psychology, 70*, 1170–1182.

Dienstmann, G. (2018). *Practical meditation: A simple step-by-step guide*. DK.

Ditzen, B., & Heinrichs, M. (2014). Psychobiology of social support: The social dimension of stress buffering. *Restorative Neurology and Neuroscience, 32*(1), 149–162.

Domonoske, C., & Gonzalez, R. (2018). What we know: Family separation and "zero tolerance" at the border. *NPR*. Retrieved from https://www.npr.org/2018/06/19/621065383/what-we-know-family-separation-and-zero-tolerance-at-the-border

Dorn, A. V., Cooney, R. E., & Sabin, M. L. (2020). COVID-19 exacerbating inequalities in the US. *Lancet, 395*(10232), 1243–1244.

Dutton, M. A., & Rubenstein, F. L. (1995). Working with people with PTSD: Research implications. In C. R. Figley (Ed.), *Compassion fatigue: Coping with secondary traumatic stress disorder in those who treat the traumatized*. Routledge.

Dwyer, L. A. (2005). *An investigation of secondary trauma in police wives* (Unpublished doctoral dissertation). Hofstra University.

Editors of Encyclopedia Britannica. (n.d.). *Stream of consciousness* [Web article]. Retrieved from https://www.britiannica.com/art/stream-of-consciouness.

Eggiman, J. (2006). Cognitive-behavioral therapy: A case report-animal assisted therapy. *Topic in Advance Practice Nursing ejournal, 6*(3). Retrieved from http://www.tmjtexas.com/attachments/contentmanagers/199/animalassistedtherapy.pdf

Ehlers, A., & Clark, D. M. (2000). A cognitive model of posttraumatic stress disorder. *Behaviour Research and Therapy, 38*, 319–345.

Eidelson, R. J., D'Alessio, G. R., & Eidelson, J. I. (2003). The impact of September 11 on psychologists. *Professional Psychology: Research and Practice, 34*(2), 144–150.

Elkington, T. J., Cassar, S., Nelson, A. R., & Levinger, I. (2017). Psychological responses to acute aerobic, resistance, or combined exercise in health and overweight individuals: A systematic review. *Clinical Insights: Cardiology, 11*, 1–23.

Ellis, A. (1975). *A new guide to rational living*. Wilshire.

Emerson, D., & Hopper, E. (2011). *Overcoming trauma through yoga: Reclaiming your body*. North Atlantic Books.

Farrell, P. A., Gates, W. K., Maksud, M. G., & Morgan, W. P. (1982). Increases in plasma beta-endorphin/beta-lipotropin immunoreactivity after treadmill running in humans. *Journal of Applied Physiology, 52*, 1245–1249.

Figley, C. R. (1989). *Treating stress in families*. Brunner/Mazel.

Figley, C. R. (1995). *Compassion fatigue: Coping with secondary traumatic stress disorder in those who treat the traumatized*. Routledge.

Figley, C. R. (2002). Compassion fatigue: Psychotherapists' chronic lack of self-care. *Journal of Clinical Psychology, 58*(11), 1433–1441.

Figley, C. R. (2003). *Compassion fatigue: An introduction*. https://www.academia.edu/2258985/Compassion_fatigue_An_intorduction?email_work_card=view-paper

Figley, C. R., & Figley, K. R. (2009). Stemming the tide of trauma systemically: The role of family therapy. *The Australian and New Zealand Journal of Family Therapy, 30*(3), 173–183.

Figley, C. R., & Kiser, L. (2013). *Helping traumatized families* (2nd ed.). Routledge.

Figley, C. R., & Ludick, M. (2017). Secondary traumatization and compassion fatigue. In S. Gold (Ed.), *Handbook of trauma psychology* (Vol. 1, pp. 573–593). APA Books.

Flueckiger, L., Lieb, R., Meyer, A. H., Witthauer, C., & Mata, J. (2016). The importance of physical activity and sleep for affect on stressful days: Two intensive longitudinal studies. *Emotion, 16*, 488–497.

Foa, E. B., & Kozak, M. J. (1986). Emotional processing of fear: Exposure to corrective information. *Psychological Bulletin, 99*, 20–35.

Foa, E. B., Keane, T. M., & Friedman, M. J. (2000). *Effective treatments for PTSD*. Guilford.

Foa, E. B., Hembree, E. A., & Rothbaum, B. O. (2007). *Prolonged exposure therapy for PTSD: Emotional process of traumatic experiences-Therapist guide*. Oxford University Press.

Foreman, A., Glenn, M., Meade, B., & Wirth, O. (2017). Dogs in the workplace: A review of the benefits and potential challenges. *International Journal of Environmental Research in Public Health, 14*(5), 498–519.

Fortylow, A. L. (2011). Integrating yoga and psychotherapy: A complementary treatment for Anxiety and depression. *Canadian Journal of Counseling and Psychotherapy, 45*, 132–150.

Fox, J. H., Burkle, F. M., Jr., Bass, J., Pia, F. A., Epstein, J. L., & Markenson, D. (2012). The effectiveness of psychological first aid as a disaster intervention tool: Research analyses of peer-reviewed literature from 1990–2010. *Disaster Medicine and Public Health Preparedness, 6*, 247–252.

Frankl, V. E. (1963). *Man's search for meaning*. Pocket Books.

Freud, A., & Burlingham, D. (1942). *War and children.* Report 12 in the writings of Anna Freud (Vol. 3). International Universities Press.

Freudenberger, H. J. (1974). Staff burnout. *Journal of Social Issues, 30*(1), 159–165.

Gallegos, A. M., Crean, H. F., Pigeon, W. R., & Heffner, K. L. (2017). Meditation and Yoga for posttraumatic stress disorder: A meta-analytic review of randomized controlled trials. *Clinical Psychology Review, 58*, 115–124.

Garbe, A., Ogurlul, U., Logan, N., & Cook, P. (2020). COVID-19 and remote learning: Experiences of parents with children during the pandemic. *American Journal of Qualitative Research, 4*(3), 45–65.

Garbern, S. C., Ebbeling, L. G., & Bartels, S. A. (2016). A systematic review of health outcomes among disaster and humanitarian responders. *Prehospital and Disaster Medicine, 31*(6), 635–642.

Gasperez, R., Nawijn, L., Lamers, F., & Pennijx, B. W. J. H. (2018). Patients with anxious depression: Overview of prevalence, pathophysiology, and impact on course and treatment outcome. *Current Opinion in Psychiatry, 31*(1), 17–25.

Gentry, J. E., Baggerly, J., & Baranowsky, A. (2004). Training-as-treatment: effectiveness of the certified compassion fatigue specialist training. *International Journal of Emergency Mental Health, 6*, 147–155.

Germer, C. K. (2005). Mindfulness. What is it? What does it matter? In C. Germer, R. Siegel, & R. Fulton (Eds.), *Mindfulness and psychotherapy* (pp. 3–27). Guildford.

Germer, C. K., Siegel, R. D., & Fulton, P. R. (2005). *Mindfulness and psychotherapy*. Guilford.

Gilbert-Eliot, T. (2020). *Healing secondary trauma: Proven strategies for caregivers and professionals to manage stress, anxiety, and compassion fatigue*. Rockridge Press.

Ginsburgh, Y. (2006). *What you need to know about Kabbalah*. Gal Einai.

Greinacher, A., Derezza-Greeven, C., Herzog, W., & Nikendei, C. (2019). Secondary traumatization in first responders: A systematic review. *European, Journal of Psychotraumatology, 10*(1), 1–24.

Gupta, S. (2020). *Keep sharp: Build a better brain at any age*. Simon and Schuster.

Haddock, C. K., Poston, W. S. C., Jahnke, S. A., & Jitnarin, N. (2017). Alcohol use and problem drinking among women firefighters. *Women's Health Issues, 27*(6), 632–638.

Haglund, M. E. M., Nestadt, P. S., Cooper, N. S., Southwick, S. M., & Charney, D. S. (2007). Psychobiological mechanisms of resilience: Relevance to prevention and treatment of stress-related psychopathology. *Development and Psychopathology, 19*(3), 889–920.

Hajar, R. (2015). Animal assisted therapy. *Heart Views, 16*(2), 70–71.

Hannah, B., & Woolgar, M. (2018). Secondary trauma and compassion fatigue in foster carers. *Clinical Child Psychology and Psychiatry, 23*(4), 629–643.

Harris, C. J. (1995). Sensory-based therapy for crisis counselors. In C. Figley (Ed.), *Compassion fatigue: Coping with secondary traumatic stress disorder in those who treat the traumatized.* Routledge.

Harrison, P. (2018). *28 different types of yoga and their benefits.* Retrieved January 15, 2022, from https://www.thedailymeditation.com/yoga-types

Hart, L. A., Zasloff, R. I., Bryson, S., & Christensen, S. L. (2000). The role of police dogs as companions and working partners. *Psychological Reports, 86*(1), 190–202.

Hatfield, E., Cacioppo, J. T., & Rapson, R. L. (1994). *Emotional contagion.* Cambridge University Press.

Hayes, S. C., Follette, V. M., & Linehan, M. N. (Eds.). (2004). *Mindfulness and acceptance: Expanding the cognitive-behavioral tradition.* Guilford.

Hayes, S. C., Strosahl, K. D., & Wilson, G. (2016). *Acceptance and commitment therapy: The process and practice of mindful change.* Spiegel and Grau.

Herman, J. L. (1992). *Trauma and recovery.* Basic Books.

Hickok, G. (2009). Eight problems for the mirror neuron theory of action understanding in monkeys and humans. *Journal of Cognitive Neuroscience, 21*(7), 1229–1243.

Hilton, L., Maher, A. H., Colaiaco, B., Apayden, E., Sorbero, M. E., Booth, M., et al. (2017). Meditation for posttraumatic stress: Systematic review and meta-analysis. *Psychological Trauma: Theory, Research, Practice, and Policy, 9*, 453–460.

History.com Editors (2020). *Sandra Bland dies in jail after traffic stop confrontation.* Retrieved from https://www.history.com/this-day-in history/sandra-bland-dies-in-jail

Hofferth, S. L. (2009). Changes in American children's time 1997–2003. *Electronic International Journal of Time Use Research, 11*, 26–47.

Hoffman, M. L. (1975). Developmental synthesis of affect and cognition and its interplay for altruistic motivation. *Developmental Psychology, 11*, 607–622.

Hoffman, M. L. (1988). Moral development. In M. Bronstein & M. Lamb (Eds.), *Developmental psychology: An advanced textbook* (pp. 497–548). Erlbaum.

Holter, M. C., Teague, G. B., & Bybee, D. (2003). Fidelity criteria: Development, measurement, and validation. *American Journal of Evaluation, 2*(3), 315–340.

Hooper, S. I., Murray, S. L., Ferrara, L. R., & Singleton, J. K. (2018, June). Effectiveness of diaphragmatic breathing on physiological and psychological stress in adults: A quantitative and systematic review protocol. *JBI Database of Systematic Reviews and Implementation Reports, 16*(6), 1367–1374.

Horn, A., Ostwald, D., Reisert, M., & Blankenburg, F. (2014). The structural-Functional connectome and the default mode network of the human brain. *NeuroImage, 102*, 142–151.

House, J. S., Landis, K. R., & Umberson, D. (1988). Social relationships and health. *Science, 241*(4865), 540–545.

Hrdy, S. B. (2011). *Mothers and others: The evolutionary origins of mutual understanding.* Harvard University Press.

Huck, L. G., & Burk, R. L. (2019). *Military veterinary services.* Office of the Surgeon General. Borden Institute, U.S. Army Medical Department Center and School, Health Readiness Center of Excellence.

Hydon, S., Wong, M., Langley, A. K., Stein, B. D., & Kataoka, S. H. (2015). Preventing secondary traumatic stress in educators. *Child and Adolescent Psychiatric Clinics of North America, 24*(2), 319–313.

Hytten, K., & Hasle, A. (1989). Firefighters: A study of stress and coping. *ACTA Psychiatry-Scandinavia Supplement, 355*, 50–55.

Ives, N. (2016). The experience of law enforcement officers when working with a K9: Social support, attachment, and stress buffering [ProQuest information & learning]. In *Dissertation abstracts international section A: Humanities and social science* (Vol. 76, Issue 9-A(E)).

Jacobson, E. (1938). *Progressive muscle relaxation.* University of Chicago Press.

Jamison, K. R. (1999). *Night falls fast: Understanding suicide*. Knoph.

Jenkins, S., & Baird, S. (2002). Secondary traumatic stress and vicarious trauma: A validation study. *Journal of Traumatic Stress, 15*, 423–432.

Johnson, R. A., Albright, D. L., Marzolf, J. R., Bibbo, J. L., Yaglom, H. D., Crowder, S. M., et al. (2018). Effects of therapeutic horseback riding on post-traumatic stress disorder in military veterans. *Military Medical Research, 5*, 3.

Jung, C. (1966). Psychology of the transference. In *The practice of psychotherapy* (Bollingen series) (Vol. 16). Princeton University Press.

Kabat-Zinn, J. (1994). *Wherever you go, there you are: Mindfulness meditation in everyday life*. Hyperion.

Kabat-Zinn, J. (2003). Mindfulness-based interventions in context: Past, present, and future. *Clinical Psychology: Science and Practice, 10*, 144–156.

Kabat-Zinn, J. (2005). *Coming to our senses: Healing ourselves and the world through mindfulness*. Hyperion.

Kaley-Isley, L. C., Petersen, J., Fischer, C., & Petersen, E. (2010). Yoga as a complementary for children and adolescents: A guide for clinicians. *Psychiatry, 7*, 20–32.

Kassai, S. C., & Motta, R. W. (2006). An investigation of the spread of potential Holocaust-related secondary traumatization to the third generation. *International Journal of Emergency Mental Health, 8*(1), 35–47.

Kellerman, N. (2001). Psychopathology in children of Holocaust survivors: A review of the research literature. *Israeli Journal of Psychiatry and Related Sciences, 38*, 36–46.

Kent de Grey, R. G., Uchino, B. N., Trettevik, R., Cronan, S., & Hogan, J. (2018). Social support. In H. S. Friedman (Ed.), *Oxford biographies* (pp. 189–214). Oxford University Press.

Kim, S. H., Schnieder, S. M., Kravitz, L., Mermier, C., & Burge, M. R. (2013). Mind-body practices for posttraumatic stress disorder. *Journal of Investigative Medicine, 61*, 827–834.

Kirby, R., Shakespeare-Finch, J., & Palk, G. (2011). Adaptive and maladaptive coping strategies predict posttrauma outcomes in ambulance personnel. *Traumatology, 17*(4), 25–34.

Kirkwood, G., Rampes, J., Tuffrey, V., Richardson, J., & Pilkington, K. (2005). Yoga for anxiety: A systematic review of the research evidence. *British Journal of Sports Medicine, 39*, 884–891.

Kishidda, M., & Elavsky, S. (2015). Daily physical activity enhances resilient resources for symptom management of middle-aged women. *Health Psychology, 34*, 756–764.

Knafo, A., Zahn-Waxler, C., Van Hulle, C., Robinson, J. L., & Rhee, S. H. (2008). The development of origins of a disposition toward empathy: Genetic and environmental contributions. *Emotion, 8*(6), 737–752.

Kogan, L. R., Rishniw, M., Hellyer, P. W., & Schoenfeld-Tacher, R. (2018). Veterinarians' experiences with near misses and adverse events. *Journal of the American Veterinary Medical Association, 252*(5), 586–595.

Kubler-Ross, E., & Kessler, D. (2014). *On grief and grieving: Finding the meaning of grief through the five stages of loss*. Simon and Shuster.

Lanning, B. A., Wilson, A. L., Woelk, R., & Beaujean, A. A. (2018). Therapeutic horseback riding as a complementary intervention for military service members with PTSD. *Human-Animal Interaction Bulletin, 6*(2), 58–82.

Levenson, R. W., & Ruef, A. M. (1992). Empathy: A physiological substrate. *Journal of Personality and Social Psychology, 38*, 16–30.

Levine, P. (2010). *In an unspoken voice: How the body releases trauma and restores goodness*. North Atlantic Books.

Li, A. W., & Goldsmith, A. W. (2012). The effects of yoga on anxiety and stress. *Alternative Medicine Review, 17*, 21–35.

Libov, B. G., Nevid, J. S., Pelcovitz, D., & Carmony, T. M. (2002). Posttraumatic stress symptomology in mothers of pediatric cancer survivors. *Psychology and Health, 19*, 501–511.

Lin, T. W., & Kuo, Y. M. (2013). Exercise benefits brain function: The monoamine connection. *Brain Sciences, 3*(1), 39–53.

Linehan, M. M. (1993). *Cognitive and behavioral treatment for borderline personality disorder*. Guilford Press.

Liu, N., Zhang, F., Wei, C., Jia, Y., Shang, Z., Sun, L., et al. (2020). Prevalence and predictors of PTSS during COVID-19 outbreak in China's hardest hit areas: Gender differences matter. *Psychiatry Research*, 112921.

Lombardo, M. (2005). *Secondary trauma in individuals exposed to a person with a serious medical illness* (Unpublished doctoral dissertation). Hofstra University.

Lombardo, K. (2007). *Secondary trauma in children of parents with mental illness* (Unpublished doctoral dissertation). Hofstra University.

Longacre, M., Dilbrt-Highfield, E., Lama, P., & Grodin, M. A. (2012). Complementary and alternative medicine in the treatment of refugees and survivors of torture: A review and proposal for action. *Torture, 22*, 38–57.

Lopez-Zeron, G., & Blow, A. (2017). The role of relationships and families in healing from trauma. *Journal of Family Therapy, 39*, 580–597.

Ludick, M. (2013). *Analyses of experiences of vicarious traumatization in short-term insurance claims workers* (Unpublished doctoral dissertation). University of the Witwatersrand.

Lupien, S. J., McEwen, B. S., Gunnar, M. R., & Hein, C. (2009). Effects of stress throughout the lifespan on the brain, behaviour and cognition. *Nature Reviews Neuroscience, 10*, 434–445.

Macy, R. J., Jones, E., Graham, L. M., & Roach, L. (2018). Yoga for trauma and related mental health problems: A meta-review with clinical and service recommendations. *Trauma, Violence, and Abuse, 19*(1), 1–37.

Marmar, C. R., McCaslin, S. E., Metzler, T. J., Best, S., Weiss, D. S., et al. (2006). Predictors of posttraumatic stress in police and other first responders. *Annals of the New York Academy of Sciences, 1071*, 1–18.

Martinsen, E. W. (1987). The role of exercise in the treatment of depression. *Stress Medicine, 3*, 93–100.

Martinsen, E. W., Hoffarat, A., & Solberg, O. (1989). Comparing aerobic and nonaerobic forms of exercise in the treatment of clinical depression: A randomized trial. *Comparative Psychiatry, 30*, 324–331.

Maslach, C. (1976). Burn-out. *Human Behavior, 5*(9), 16–22.

Maslach, C., & Leiter, M. (1997). *The truth about burnout: How organizations cause personal stress and what to do about it*. Josey-Bass.

Masserman, J. H., Wechkin, S., & Terris, W. (1964). 'Altruistic' behavior in rhesus monkeys. *The American Journal of Psychiatry, 121*(6), 584–585.

Mayou, R. A., Ehlers, A., & Hobbs, M. (2000). Psychological debriefing for road traffic accident victims. *British Journal of Psychiatry, 176*, 589–593.

McCafferty, F., Domingo, G., & McCafferty, E. (1990). PTSD in the police officer: Paradigm of occupational stress. *Southern Medical Journal, 83*, 543–547.

McCann, I. L., & Pearlman, L. A. (1990). Vicarious traumatization: A framework for understanding the psychological effects of working with victims. *Journal of Traumatic Stress, 3*(1), 131–149.

Mead, E. (2020, January 17). *The history and origin of the word meditation*. Retrieved from https://positivepsychology.com/history-of-meditation/

Mehta, P., & Sharma, M. (2010). Yoga as a complementary therapy for clinical depression. *Complementary Health Practice Review, 15*, 156–170.

Michenbaum, D. (1985). *Stress inoculation training*. Pergamon Press.

Miller, B., & Sprang, G. (2017). A components based practice and supervision model for reducing compassion fatigue by affecting clinician experience. *Traumatology, 23*(2), 153–164.

Miller, R. E., Banks, J. H., Jr., & Ogawa, N. (1963). Role of facial expression in 'cooperative-avoidance conditioning' in monkeys. *Journal of Abnormal and Social Psychology, 67*(1), 24–30. https://doi.org/10.1037/h0044018

Mitchell, J. (1983). When disaster strike. The critical incident stress debriefing process. *Journal of Emergency Medical Services, 22*, 87–93.

Mitchell, J. (2011). Collateral damage in disaster workers. *International Journal of Emergency Mental Health and Resilience, 13*(2), 95–120.

Mitchell, J. T., & Everly, G. S. (1997). Scientific evidence for CISM. *Journal of Emergency Services, 22*, 87–93.

Mitchell, J. T., & Everly, G. S. (2000). Critical incident stress management and critical incident stress debriefings: Evolutions, effects, and outcomes. In B. Raphael & J. Wilson (Eds.), *Psychological debriefing: Theory, practice and evidence* (pp. 71–90). Cambridge University Press.

Molnar, B. E., Sprang, G., Killian, K. D., Gottfried, R., Emery, V., & Bride, B. E. (2017). Advancing science and practice for vicarious traumatization/secondary traumatic stress: A research agenda. *Traumatology, 23*(2), 129–142.

Morina, N., Wicherts, J. M., Lobbrecht, J., & Priebe, S. (2014). Remission from post-traumatic stress disorder in adults: A systematic review and meta-analysis of long-term outcome studies. *Clinical Psychology Review, 34*, 249–255.

Motta, R. W. (2005). Secondary trauma in children: A call for research. *The School Psychologist, 59*(3), 108–112.

Motta, R. W. (2015). Trauma, PTSD, and secondary trauma in children and adolescents. In R. Flanagan (Ed.), *Cognitive and behavioral interventions in the schools* (pp. 67–84). Springer.

Motta, R. W. (2018). The role of exercise in reducing PTSD and negative emotional states. In S. G. Taukeni (Ed.), *Psychology of health-biopsychosocial approach*. IntechOpen.

Motta, R. W. (2020). *Alternative therapies for PTSD: The science of mind-body Treatments*. American Psychological Association.

Motta, R. W. (2021). *Altered: A trauma and PTSD casebook*. Kindle Direct Publishing.

Motta, R. W., Kefer, J. M., Hertz, M. D., & Hafeez, S. (1999). Initial evaluation of the Secondary trauma questionnaire. *Psychological Reports, 85*, 997–1002.

Motta, R. W., Hafeez, S., Sciancalepore, R., & Diaz, A. B. (2001). Discriminant validation of the secondary trauma scale. *Journal of Psychotherapy in Independent Practice, 24*, 17–24.

Mulcahy, K. A. (1988). *Beck's cognitive therapy and aerobic exercise for the treatment of depression* (Unpublished doctoral dissertation). Hofstra University. ProQuest Dissertations Publishing, 9822257.

National Center for Complementary and Alternative Medicine. (2014). *Yoga*. National Institutes of Health, U.S. Department of Health and Human Services. Retrieved from http://nccam.nih.gov.ezproxy.hofstra.edu/health/yoga

Neff, K. D., Kilpatrick, K., & Rude, S. (2007). Self-compassion and its link to adaptive psychological functioning. *Journal of Research in Personality, 4*(1), 908–916.

Neill, J. T. (2003). Reviewing and benchmarking adventure therapy outcomes: Applications of meta-analysis. *Journal of Experimental Education, 25*, 316–321.

Nelson, B. S., & Wampler, K. S. (2000). Systemic effects of trauma in clinic couples: An exploratory study of secondary trauma resulting from childhood abuse. *Journal of Marital and Family Therapy, 26*, 171–184.

Nieforth, L. O., & O'Haire, M. E. (2020). The role of pets in managing uncertainty from COVID-19. *Psychological Trauma: Theory, Research, Practice, and Policy, 12*(S1), S345–S246.

Nightingale, F. (1969). *Notes on nursing: What it is and what it is not*. Dover.

Nolen-Hoeksema, S., Wisco, B. E., & Lyubromirsky, S. (2008). Rethinking rumination. *Perspectives on Psychological Science, 3*, 400–424.

Norcross, J. C. (2000). Psychotherapist self-care: Practitioner-tested, research-informed strategies. *Professional Psychology: Research and Practice, 31*(60), 710–713.

NPR.org, Westervelt, E. (2021, June). *Cops say low morale and department scrutiny are driving them away from the job.*

O'Haire, M. E., & Rodriguez, K. E. (2018). Preliminary efficacy of service dogs as a complementary treatment for posttraumatic stress disorder in military members and veterans. *Journal of Consulting and Clinical Psychology, 86*, 179–188.

O'Haire, M. E., Guerin, N. A., & Kirkham, A. C. (2015). Animal assisted intervention for trauma: A systematic literature review. *Frontiers in Psychology, 6*, 121.

Odou, N., & Brinker, J. (2014). Exploring the relationship between rumination, self-compassion, and mood. *Self and Identity, 13*(4), 449–459.

Oginska-Bulik, N., Guroiec, P. J., Michalska, P., & Kedra, E. (2021). Prevalence and predictors of secondary traumatic stress symptoms in health care professionals working with trauma victims: A cross-sectional study. *PLoS One, 16*(2), 1–19.

Osborne, K. R., Duprey, E. B., O'Brien Caugh, M., & Oshri, A. (2021). Parents' maltreatment history, dimension of emotional regulation, and connection to offspring self-regulation: A sex specific transmission pathway. *Journal of Psychopathology and Behavioral Assessment*. https://doi.org/10.1007/s10862-021-09881-4

Parish-Plass, N. (2008). Animal-assisted therapy with children suffering from insecure attachment due to abuse and neglect: A method to lower the risk of intergenerational transmission of abuse? *Clinical Child Psychology and Psychiatry, 13*(1), 7–30.

Patki, G., Li, L., Allam, F., Solanki, N., Dao, A. T., Alkadhi, K., & Salim, S. (2014). Moderate treadmill exercise rescues anxiety and depression-like behavior as well as memory impairment in a rat model of posttraumatic stress disorder. *Physiology and Behavior, 130*, 47–53.

Pearlman, L. A., & Saakvitne, K. W. (1995). Treating therapists with vicarious traumatization and secondary traumatic stress disorders. In C. Figley (Ed.), *Compassion fatigue: Coping with secondary traumatic stress disorder in those who treat the traumatized* (pp. 150–177). Routledge.

Pendry, P., Smith, A. N., & Roeter, S. M. (2014). Randomized trial examines the effects of equine facilitated learning on adolescents' basal cortisol levels. *Human-Animal Interaction Bulletin, 2*(1), 80–93.

Pennebaker, J. W. (1997). Writing about emotional experiences as a therapeutic process. *Psychological Science, 8*, 162–166.

Perlstein, R., & Motta, R. W. (2012). An Investigation of potential Holocaust-related secondary trauma in the third generation. *Traumatology, 19*(2), 95–106. https://doi.org/10.1177/153765612449659

Pert, C. B. (1999). *Molecules of emotion: The science behind mind-body medicine*. Scribner.

Pert, C. B., Ruff, M. R., Weber, R. J., & Herkenham, M. (1985). Neuropeptides and their receptors: A psychosomatic network. *Journal of Immunology, 135*, 820–826.

Phipps, A. B., & Byrne, M. K. (2003). Brief interventions for secondary trauma: Review and recommendations. *Stress and Health, 19*, 139–147.

Pitman, R. K. (1989). Post-traumatic stress disorder, hormones, and memory. *Biological Psychiatry, 26*(3), 221–223.

Prati, G., Pietrantoni, L., & Cicognani, E. (2010). Self-efficacy moderates the relationship between stress appraisal and quality of life among rescue workers. *Anxiety, Stress, & Coping: An International Journal, 23*, 463–470.

Preston, J. D., O'Neal, J. H., & Talaga, M. C. (2002). *Handbook of clinical psychopharmacology for therapists* (3rd ed.). New Harbinger.

Quevillon, R. P., Gray, B. L., Erickson, S. E., Gonzalez, E. D., & Jacobs, G. G. (2016). Helping the helpers: Assisting staff and volunteer workers before, during, and after disaster relief operations. *Journal of Clinical Psychology, 72*(12), 1348–1363.

Rauvola, R. S., Dulce, M. V., & Lavigne, K. N. (2019). Compassion fatigue, secondary traumatic stress, and vicarious traumatization: A qualitative review and research agenda. *Occupational Health Science, 3*, 297–336.

Remer, R., & Ferguson, R. A. (1998). Treating traumatized partners: Producing secondary survivors of PTSD. In C. R. Figley (Ed.), *Burnout in families: The systematic costs of caring*. CRC Press.

Resick, P. A. (2001). *Cognitive processing therapy: Generic version*. University of Missouri: St. Lewis.

Reyes, H. (2007). The worst scars are in the mind: Psychological torture. *International Review of the Red Cross, 89*, 591–617.

Richards, D. A. (2009). A field study of critical incident stress debriefing versus critical incident stress management. *Journal of Mental Health, 10*(3), 351–362.

Riley, K. E., & Park, C. L. (2015). How does yoga reduce stress? A systematic review of mechanisms of change and guide to future inquiry. *Health Psychology Review, 9*, 379–396.

Rizzolatti, G., & Fadiga, L. (1999). Resonance behaviors and motor neurons. *Italieenes de Biologie, 137*(2–2), 85–100.

Robbins, J. (2020, June 9). Ecopsychology: How immersion in nature benefits your health. *Yale Environment, 360.* https://360-yale.edu.features.ecopsychology-how-in-nature-benefits-your-health

Roden-Foreman, J. W., Bennett, M. M., Rainey, E. E., Garrett, J. S., Powers, M. B., & Warren, A. M. (2017). Secondary traumatic stress in emergency medicine clinicians. *Cognitive Behavior Therapy, 46*(6), 522–532.

Rodriguez, H., Ryan, S., Rowan, A. B., & Foy, D. W. (1996). Posttraumatic stress disorder in a clinical sample of adult survivors of childhood sexual abuse. *Child Abuse & Neglect, 20*, 943–952.

Rosenheck, R. (1986). Impact of posttraumatic stress disorder or World War II on the next generation. *Journal of Nervous and Mental Disease, 174*(6), 319–327.

Rosenheck, R., & Nathan, P. (1985). Secondary traumatization in children of Vietnam Veterans. *Hospital and Community Psychiatry, 36*(5), 538–539.

Rudofossi, D. (2007). *Working with traumatized police officer-patients: A clinical guide complex PTSD syndromes in public safety professionals*. Baywood.

Salston, M. D., & Figley, C. R. (2003). Secondary traumatic stress effects of working with survivors of criminal victimization. *Journal of Traumatic Stress, 16*(2), 167–174.

Salzberg, S. (1995). *Lovingkindness: The revolutionary art of happiness*. Shambhala.

Schlenger, W. E., Caddell, J. M., Ebert, L., Jordan, B. K., Rourke, K. M., Wilson, D., et al. (2002). Psychological reactions to terrorist attacks: Findings from the national study of Americans' reactions to September 11. *JAMA, 288*, 581–588. https://doi.org/10.1001/jama.288.5.581

Schwarzmuller-Eber, G., Meier, M., Stummer, H., & Kundi, M. (2021). Recreational horseback riding and its association with physical, mental, and social wellbeing and perceived health. *Anthrozoös, 34*(5), 685–706.

Sciancalepore, R. S., & Motta, R. W. (2004). Gender related correlates of posttraumatic stress disorder in A World Trade Center Sample. *International Journal of Emergency Mental Health, 6*(1), 15–31.

Sexton, L. (1999). Vicarious traumatization of counsellors and the effects on their workplaces. *British Journal of Guidance and Counseling, 27*, 393–403.

Shakespeare-Finch, J., Rees, A., & Armstrong, D. (2015). Social support, self-efficacy, trauma and well-being in emergency medical dispatchers. *Social Indicators Research, 123*, 549–565.

Shapiro, F. (2001). *Eye movement desensitization and reprocessing: Basic principles, protocols, and procedures* (2nd ed.). Guilford.

Shivakumar, G., Anderson, E. H., Suris, A. M., & North, C. S. (2017). Exercise of PTSD in women veterans: A proof-of-concept study. *Military Medicine, 182*, e1809–e1814.

Shulz, R., Beach, S. R., Czaja, S. J., Martire, L. M., & Monin, J. K. (2020). Family caregiving for older adults. *Annual Review of Psychology, 71*, 635–659.

Smaga, I., Bystrowska, B., Gawlinski, D., Przegalinski, R., & Filip, M. (2014). The endocannaboinid/endovanilloid system and depression. *Current Neuropharmacology, 12*, 462–474.

Smith, A. (1759). 1948 The theory of moral sentiments. In H. Schneider (Ed.), *Adam Smith's moral and political philosophy* (pp. 3–277). Hafner.

Smith, A. (1950). *An inquiry into the nature and causes of the wealth of nations* (2 Vols., 6th ed). Edited, with an introduction, notes, marginal summary, and an enlarged index by Edwin Cannan. Methuen (Original work published 1776).

Smith, A. (1976). *The theory of moral sentiments*. Clarendon Press (Original work published 1759).

Smith, E. (2018, December 11). *What is thought stopping? Therapy, techniques, exercises, healthyplace*. https://www.healthyplace.com/self-help/positivity/what-is-thought-stopping-therapy-techniques-exercises

Smolkovic, I. (2012). Attachment to pets and interpersonal relationships. *Journal of European Psychological Studies, 3*, 15–23.

Sobo, E. J., Eng, B., & Kassity-Krish, N. (2006). Canine visitation (pet) therapy: Pilot data on decreases in child pain perception. *Journal of Holistic Nursing, 24*(1), 51–57.

Soler, J., Cebolla, A., Feliu-Soler, A., Demarzo, M. M. P., Pascual, J. C., Banos, R., & Garcia-Campayo, J. (2014). Relationship between meditative practice and self-reported mindfulness: The Mindsens composite index. *PLoS One, 9*, e86622. https://doi.org/10.1371/journal.pone.0086622

Southwick, S. M., Vythilingam, M., & Charney, D. S. (2005). The psychobiology of depression and resilience to stress: Implications for prevention and treatment. *Annual Review of Clinical Psychology, 1*, 255–291.

Sprang, G., Clark, J. J., & Whitt-Woosley, A. (2007). Compassion fatigue, compassion Satisfaction, and burnout: Factors impacting a professional's quality of life. *Journal of Loss and Trauma, 12*, 259–280.

Stamm, B. H. (2010). *The concise ProQOL manual*. ProQOL. Org.

Stanley, I. H., Hom, M. A., Kimbrel, N. A., & Joiner, T. E. (2017). Differences in psychiatric symptoms and barriers to mental health care between volunteer and career firefighters. *Psychiatry Research, 247*, 236–242.

Steele, W. (1992). *Preventing self-destruction: A manual for school crisis response teams*. Learning Publications.

Stein, G. (1922). *Geography and plays*. The Four Seasons.

Stephens, C., & Long, N. (2000). Communication with police supervisors as a buffer of work-related traumatic stress. *Journal of Organizational Behavior, 21*, 407–424.

Stout, M. (2005). *The sociopath next door*. Harmony.

Strohle, A. (2009). Physical activity, exercise, depression and anxiety disorders. *Journal of Neural Transmission, 116*, 777–784.

Stroop, J. R. (1935). Studies of interference in serial verbal reaction. *Journal of Experimental Psychology, 18*, 643–662. https://doi.org/10.1037/h0054651

Sultanoff, B. A. (2001). Breath work. In Shannon (Ed.), *Handbook of complementary and alternative therapies in mental health*. Academic Press.

Suozzi, J. M., & Motta, R. W. (2004). The relationship between combat exposure and the transfer of trauma-like symptoms to offspring of veterans. *Traumatology, 10*(1), 17–37.

Taylor, A. J. W., & Fraser, A. G. (1982). The stress of post-disaster body handling and victim identification work. *Journal of Human Stress, 8*, 4–12.

Teasdale, J. D., Segal, Z. V., Williams, J. M., Ridgeway, V. A., Soulsby, J. M., & Lau, M. A. (2000). Prevention of relapse/recurrence in major depression by mindfulness-based cognitive therapy. *Journal of Consulting and Clinical Psychology, 68*, 615–623.

Tedeschi, R. G., & Calhoun, L. G. (1996). The posttraumatic growth inventory: Measuring the positive legacy of trauma. *Journal of Traumatic Stress, 9*, 455–471.

Tedeschi, R. G., & Calhoun, L. G. (2004). *Posttraumatic growth: Conceptual foundations and empirical evidence*. Lawrence Erlbaum.

Tedeschi, P., & Jenkins, M. A. (2019). *Transforming trauma: Resilience and healing through our connections with animals*. Purdue University Press (Knowledge Unlatched Open Access Edition).

Tehrani, N. (2016). Extraversion, neuroticism, and secondary trauma in internet child abuse investigators. *Occupational Medicine, 66*(5), 403–407.

Telles, S., Singh, N., & Balkrishna, A. (2012). Managing mental health disorders resulting from trauma through yoga: A review. *Depression Research and Treatment, 2012*, 1–9.

Terr, L. (1981). Forbidden games-Post-traumatic child's play. *Journal of the American Academy of Child Psychiatry, 20*, 741–760.

Terrill, W., & Reisig, M. D. (2003). Neighborhood context and police use of force. *Journal of Research in Crime and Delinquency, 40*(3), 291–321.

Thieleman, K., & Caccciatore, J. (2014). Witness to suffering: Mindfulness and compassion fatigue among traumatic bereavement volunteers and professionals. *Social Work, 59*, 34–41.

Tomporowski, P. D., Davis, C. D., Miller, P. H., & Naglieri, J. A. (2008). Exercise and children's intelligence, cognition, and academic achievement. *Educational Psychology Review, 20*, 111–131.

Treleaven, D. A. (2018). *Trauma sensitive mindfulness*. Norton.

Turlow, R. G. (2017). *Mindfulness skills for trauma and PTSD: Practices for recovery and resilience*. Norton.

Uebelacker, L. A., Epstein-Lobow, G., Gaudiano, B. A., Tremont, G., Battle, C. L., & Miller, I. W. (2010). Hatha yoga for depression: Critical review of the evidence, efficacy, plausible mechanisms of action, and direction for future research. *Journal of Psychiatric Practice, 16*, 22–33.

Van den Berg, A. E. (2017). From green space to green prescriptions: Challenges and opportunities for research and practice. *Frontiers in Psychology, 8*, 8–11.

van den Bosch, M. A., & Depledge, M. H. (2015). Healthy people with nature in mind. *BMC Public Health, 15*, 1252.

van der Kolk, B. A. (2006). Clinical implications of neuroscience research in PTSD. *Annals of the New York Academy of Sciences, 1071*, 277–293.

van der Kolk, B. E. (2014). *The body keeps the score: Brain, mind, and body in the healing of trauma*. Viking Press.

van Dernoot Lipsky, L. (2009). *Trauma Stewardship: An everyday guide to caring for self while caring for others*. Berrett-Koehler Publishers.

van IJzendoorn, M. H., Bakermans-Kranenburg, & Sagi Schwartz, A. (2003). Are children of Holocaust survivors less well-adapted? A meta-analytic investigation of secondary traumatization. *Journal of Traumatic Stress, 16*(5), 459–469.

Vujanovic, A. A., Niles, B., Pietrefesa, A., Schmertz, S. K., & Potter, C. M. (2013). Mindfulness in the treatment of posttraumatic stress disorder among military veterans. *Spirituality in Clinical Practice, 1*, 15–25.

Waddell, C., & Godderis, R. (2005). Rethinking evidence-based practice for children's mental health. *Evidence-Based Mental Health, 8*, 60–63.

Wasco, S. M., & Campbell, R. (2002). Emotional reactions of rape victim advocates: A multiple case study of anger and fear. *Psychology of Women Quarterly, 26*(2), 120–130.

Waters, L.M. (2018). *Factors influencing the vicarious effects of trauma in hotline volunteers* (Unpublished doctoral dissertation). Hofstra University.

Watkins, A, Rothfeld, M., Rashbaum, W. K., & Rosenthal, B. M. (2020, April 27). Top E.R. doctor who treated virus patients dies by suicide. *The New York Times*. https://www.nytimes.com/2020/04/27/nyregion/new-york-city-doctor-suicide-coronavirus.html

Waysman, M., Mikulinger, M., Solomon, Z., & Weisenberg, M. (1993). Secondary traumatization among wives of posttraumatic combat veterans: A family typology. *Journal of Family Psychology, 7*, 104–118.

Weintraub, A. (2012). *Yoga skills for therapists: Effective practices for mood management*. Norton.

Weiss, D. S., & Marmar, C. R. (1997). The impact of event scale-revised. In J. P. Wilson & T. M. Keans (Eds.), *Assessing psychological trauma and PTSD* (pp. 399–411). Guilford Press.

White, M. P., Pahl, S., Wheeler, B. W., Depledge, M. H., & Fleming, L. E. (2017). Natural environments and subjective wellbeing: Different types of exposure are associated are associated with different aspects of wellbeing. *Health & Place, 45*, 77–84.

Whitebird, R. R., Kreitzer, M. J., Crain, A. L., Lewis, B. A., Hanson, L. R., & Enstad, C. J. (2012). Mindfulness-based stress reduction for family care givers: A randomized controlled trial. *The Gerontologist, 53*(4), 676–686.

Whitten, M. R. (2008). Some questions about attachment theory implications for the development of mind in infancy. *The Annual of Psychoanalysis, 36*, 216–229.

Whitworth, J. W., Craft, L. L., Dunsiger, S. L., & Ciccolo, J. T. (2017). Direct and indirect effects of exercise on posttraumatic stress disorder symptoms: A longitudinal study. *General Hospital Psychiatry, 49*, 56–62.
Williams, T. (1993). Trauma in the workplace. In J. P. Wilson & B. Raphael (Eds.), *International handbook of traumatic stress and syndromes*. Plenum Press.
Williams, M. B. (1998). Treating STSD in children. In C. R. Figley (Ed.), *Burnout in families: the systemic costs of caring*. CRC Press.
Williams, F. (2017). *The nature fix*. Norton.
Williams, C. M., & Williams, T. (1987). Family therapy for Vietnam veterans. In T. Williams (Ed.), *Posttraumatic stress disorder: A handbook for clinicians* (pp. 221–231). Disabled American Veterans.
Wilson, E. O. (1984). *Biophilia*. Harvard University Press.
Wompold, B. E. (2010). The research evidence for the common factor models: A historically situated perspective. In B.L. Duncan, S.D. Miller, B.E. Wompold,& M.A. Hubble (Eds), *The heart and soul of change: Delivering what works intherapy* (pp. 49–81). American Psychological Association.
Wompold, B. E. (2015). How important are common factors in psychotherapy? An update. *World Psychiatry, 14*(3), 270–277.
Woody, R. H. (2005). The police culture: Research implications for psychological services. *Professional Psychology: Research and Practice, 36*, 525–529.
Woody, R. H. (2006). Family interventions with law enforcement officers. *American Journal of Family Therapy, 34*, 95–103.
Worden, J. W. (1991). *Grief counseling and grief therapy: A handbook for the mental health practitioner* (2nd ed.). Springer.
Wright, D. B. (2016). *Side Effects: A journey through secondary traumatic stress*. Friesen Press.
Wright, R. (2017). *Why Buddhism is true: The science and philosophy of meditation and enlightenment*. Simon & Shuster.
Yarborough, B. J. H., Stumbo, S. P., Yarborough, M. T., Owen-Smith, A., & Green, C. A. (2018). Benefits and challenges of using service dogs for veterans with posttraumatic disorder. *Psychiatric Rehabilitation Journal, 41*, 118–124.
Yoshikawa, H., & Kalil, A. (2011). The effects of parental undocumented status on the developmental contexts of young children in immigrant families. *Child Development Perspectives, 5*(4), 291–297.
Ziv, A., & Israeli, R. (1973). Effects of bombardment on the manifest anxiety level of children living in kibbutzim. *Journal of Consulting and Clinical Psychology, 40*, 187.

# Index



© The Editor(s) (if applicable) and The Author(s), under exclusive license to Springer Nature Switzerland AG 2023
R. W. Motta, *Secondary Trauma*, https://doi.org/10.1007/978-3-031-44308-4

The manufacturer's authorised representative in the EU is Springer Nature Customer Service Centre GmbH, Europaplatz 3, 69115 Heidelberg, Germany. If you have any concerns regarding our products, please contact ProductSafety@springernature.com

Printed and bound by CPI Group (UK) Ltd, Croydon, CR0 4YY
01/10/2026
02225897-0003